T0024118

Plague: A Very Short Introduction

VERY SHORT INTRODUCTIONS are for anyone wanting a stimulating and accessible way into a new subject. They are written by experts, and have been translated into more than 45 different languages.

The series began in 1995, and now covers a wide variety of topics in every discipline. The VSI library currently contains over 650 volumes—a Very Short Introduction to everything from Psychology and Philosophy of Science to American History and Relativity—and continues to grow in every subject area.

Very Short Introductions available now:

Available soon:

For more information visit our website

www.oup.com/vsi/

Paul Slack

PLAGUE

A Very Short Introduction
SECOND EDITION

OXFORD

UNIVERSITY PRESS

Great Clarendon Street, Oxford, OX2 6DP,
United Kingdom

Oxford University Press is a department of the University of Oxford.
It furthers the University's objective of excellence in research, scholarship,
and education by publishing worldwide. Oxford is a registered trade mark of
Oxford University Press in the UK and in certain other countries

© Paul Slack 2021

The moral rights of the author have been asserted

First edition published 2012
This edition published 2021

Impression: 1

All rights reserved. No part of this publication may be reproduced, stored in
a retrieval system, or transmitted, in any form or by any means, without the
prior permission in writing of Oxford University Press, or as expressly permitted
by law, by licence or under terms agreed with the appropriate reprographics
rights organization. Enquiries concerning reproduction outside the scope of the
above should be sent to the Rights Department, Oxford University Press, at the
address above

You must not circulate this work in any other form
and you must impose this same condition on any acquirer

Published in the United States of America by Oxford University Press
198 Madison Avenue, New York, NY 10016, United States of America

British Library Cataloguing in Publication Data

Data available

Library of Congress Control Number: 2020951748

ISBN 978-0-19-887111-8

Printed and bound by
CPI Group (UK) Ltd, Croydon, CR0 4YY

Links to third party websites are provided by Oxford in good faith and
for information only. Oxford disclaims any responsibility for the materials
contained in any third party website referenced in this work.

Contents

Acknowledgements

I am grateful to the many colleagues with whom I have discussed plague and plagues over the years, to Luciana O'Flaherty who first suggested this *Very Short Introduction* to me, and to others at OUP, Andrea Keegan and Jenny Nugee, who have helped me bring it to a conclusion. The anonymous readers for the Press saved me from many errors of fact and interpretation, and responsibility for those which remain is solely mine.

List of illustrations

Introduction

Anyone interested in the past knows something about plague, about
the Black Death perhaps, or the Great Plague of London—the
global pandemic of Corona-virus in 2019–20 has generated fresh
interest in epidemic disasters of that kind, and what they have to
tell us about how people responded to them. This little book is
designed for those who want to know more, and as a brief
introduction to what is now a very large, scholarly, and popular
literature accumulated around plague, much of it questioning the
identity, causes, and effects of past epidemic disasters.

My approach is that of a historian, interested in understanding
the impact of great epidemic diseases in the past and the ways in
which they have been interpreted. The conclusions (and
speculations) arising from modern medical and environmental
science will have a place, chiefly in Chapters 1–3, since they may
help to explain the incidence and effects of plague in the past
while forming a part of its cultural impact in the present. But
I have tried also, in Chapters 4–6, to explain what plague meant
for those who suffered from it in earlier centuries, for the
governments and public authorities who set out to fight it, and for
the authors, past and present, who have written about it.

The history of plague, like that of many other epidemic diseases, is
full of unexpected twists and turns, and its course is often as

difficult to explain today, with all the benefits of medical hindsight, as it was for people who experienced it then. That is part of the subject's perennial fascination. But its interest lies also in the ways in which people coped with sudden death and disease in earlier centuries and how they somehow came to terms with them. The book is arranged by themes rather than as a straightforward chronology, but I hope that it shows the important continuities in the story which can be observed over time. My aim has been to look at past pandemics of plague from a variety of standpoints, and in my final Chapter 7—on 'The lessons of histories'—to bring out what we may still have to learn from them.

Oxford, August 2020

Chapter 1
Plague: what's in a name?

Names are always important because they create identities. They are particularly important when it comes to diseases, where a name, a diagnosis, carries with it some reassurance that the phenomenon is known and understood. It may nowadays indicate its characteristic symptoms—as with 'AIDS'—or the pathogen responsible for them—as with 'HIV'—and so offer some prospect of treatment and perhaps cure. The names of diseases, and especially those of epidemic diseases, often have very long histories, however. They have sometimes been applied to past illnesses with symptoms which modern medical science has shown to be caused by more than one biological agent. Leprosy and 'the great pox' are examples.

The identity of plague is a classic case of uncertainty of this kind. It is susceptible to a variety of interpretations, and its identity has been the subject of much dispute. In its Greek and Latin origin, 'plague' meant a blow, something sudden and acute, and in general parlance it has often been employed as a generic term, applicable to almost any calamity, and to pests like locusts as well as to human and animal diseases of many kinds. The sense in which it is used in this book, and in many larger works on which this one draws, is more precise—though still sometimes contentious. 'Plague' is the word that has been used over the centuries to denote an epidemic disease of particular severity and dramatic impact, and a disease which probably always had the same causative agent, now known to have been a bacillus, *Yersinia pestis*.

Across most of its recorded history, plague has been distinguished from other epidemic diseases in two ways. First, it killed more people more quickly. In major outbreaks in European cities between the 14th and 17th centuries, it was not unusual for one-quarter of the population to die within a year (Figure 1), and it is likely that almost as many more might have been infected and then have recovered. In terms of mortality and morbidity, plague's only rivals may be the smallpox which Europeans took to the Americas after 1492 and the worldwide Spanish flu of 1918–19. Each of those disasters was undoubtedly of great historical significance, but neither has left the long written record of recurrent epidemics that allows the history of plague to be written.

The second distinguishing feature of plague, evident from that long series of records, lies in the special horrors which it inflicted on its victims and which threatened all those around them. The more elaborate descriptions, most of them surviving from the 14th century onwards, commonly refer to the extreme delirium, fever, and painful tumours of the sick, and to the putrid matter issuing from their sores, mouths, and nostrils which could contaminate anyone nearby. 'The breath is so stinking', one French physician recorded in 1666, 'that it is virtually intolerable; thus the common proverb in French is true, "one smells of plague"'. Easily sensed and identified, polluting whole cities, that cause of private suffering and collective disaster has, since at least the 6th century AD, been given the same name: plague or pestilence, *pestis* in Latin, and sometimes *the* plague or *the* pestilence.

This book will focus on the history of the disease in major epidemic form, so far as that is known, and in periods when its ravages were most pronounced, down to the first decades of the

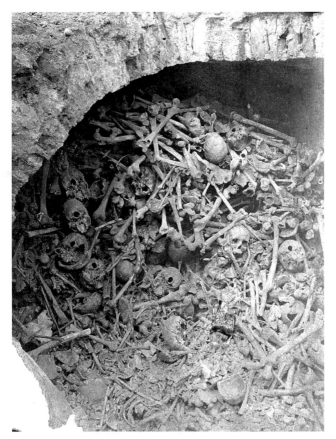

1. A London burial pit, probably in use during the plague of 1665–6.

20th century. Since the 1920s, partly thanks to public health measures and modern antibiotics, plague has been less serious as a human affliction, but it has not disappeared. It persists among animals in many parts of the world, though not in Europe, and flares up occasionally in isolated epidemics, minor in comparison with those of the past. Since 1990, however, the number of human cases has been rising. Between 1,000 and 5,000 are being reported annually to the World Health Organization, many of them in parts of Africa and Asia where there had been none for several decades, and plague is now classified as a re-emerging disease.

In its late 20th-century manifestations, plague is certainly much better understood than it has ever been. Since the 1940s, it has been the subject of extensive research, prompted in part by the possibility of its use in biological warfare or terrorism, and there are now many scientific papers and statistical studies about its prevalence, its animal reservoirs and carriers, and its clinical impact on human beings. The findings of modern medical science about plague's causes (its aetiology) and its incidence and distribution (its epidemiology) have illuminated many aspects of its history, but they have not removed all the uncertainties surrounding it. On the contrary, they have given rise to considerable debate about whether all the plagues of the past can have had the same cause as those of the present.

Plague or not?

The scientific techniques of pathology, bacteriology, and epidemiology, developed by investigators of cholera and other epidemic diseases in the 19th century, were first applied to plague when it suddenly erupted in the cities of China and India in the 1890s. The organism was first isolated in 1894, almost simultaneously, by Shibasaburo Kitasato, a Japanese pupil of Robert Koch, and Alexandre Yersin, a Swiss pupil of Pasteur, both of them working in Hong Kong (see Figure 2). It was a bacillus, then known as *Pasteurella pestis* and now called *Yersinia pestis* in Yersin's honour. From then onwards, plague was a specific entity, biologically distinguishable from diseases with other causes. Yersin showed, further, that rats were carriers of the disease, and in 1898 Paul-Louis Simond demonstrated that plague was transmitted from rodents to humans by fleas.

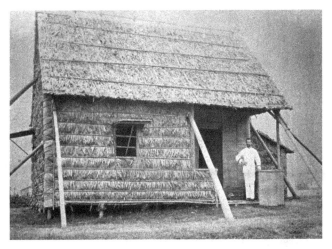

2. Alexandre Yersin outside his hut in Hong Kong, 1894.

By 1900, the classic model of urban plague had been established. It was a disease coming in from outside, from rodent reservoirs far from centres of dense human populations. Once it arrived, it was transported between cities by infected rats (on ships, for example), and was then transmitted to local rats and fleas which were sources for human infection. Investigators in China and India also established plague's typical clinical features. These include high temperatures, carbuncles at the site of the initial flea bites, and painful buboes (or swellings) at the lymph nodes, usually in the neck, groin, or armpit, which are plague's most obvious clinical symptom (see Figure 3). Death commonly occurs within three to five days of onset, and, in the absence of appropriate treatment, between 40 per cent and 60 per cent of the victims die. Later researchers distinguished other manifestations of plague, including a rare and particularly severe pneumonic variety, spread directly from person to person, without buboes and some of the other symptoms. But the predominant form of plague since the 1890s has been 'bubonic plague'.

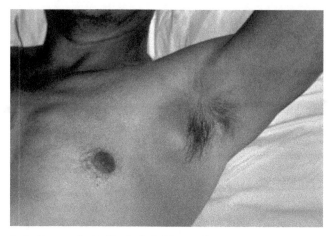

3. A plague patient with a bubo in his armpit.

Even before the 1890s, modern epidemiologists were naturally interested in the history of the diseases they studied, and new information about plague in Asia was quickly applied to earlier epidemics where the same name had been used, and especially to European epidemics, since the epidemiologists had generally been trained there. There had been European epidemics described as pestilence in Latin or Greek between the 6th and 8th centuries AD, but little was then known about them. Attention focused instead on the many plagues, chronicled in more accessible languages, which occurred between the 14th and 18th centuries. They began with the 'great pestilence' of 1347 to 1352, which has become known as the Black Death (a label first coined by Scandinavian chroniclers of the 16th century), and one of the last epidemics of plague was a famous outbreak in Marseilles in 1720. It was possible to find contemporary references to buboes in most of them—and the presence of rats and fleas in the crowded cities they affected might reasonably be assumed.

Almost immediately, however, discrepancies between modern and past plagues were identified. Not only were there scarcely any early references to fleas or even rats in association with plague. The epidemiology of the disease also appeared to be different. In the past, cases of plague had tended to cluster in family and household concentrations, but that was not obviously so in India in the 1890s. Most striking of all, between 1347 and 1352 plague spread with lethal effect across almost the whole of Europe with a speed never witnessed in modern India or China, despite modern transport facilities.

The more that was discovered about both past and more recent plagues, the more obvious the differences became. Several historians of European plagues have consequently been sceptical about their attribution to *Yersinia pestis*, and biologists have looked for alternatives which might have been at work alongside it, or even have been wholly responsible for the great mortalities evident in the historical record. None of these suggestions from outright 'plague-deniers' has commanded assent, however.

What must now be accepted is that the modern model of plague cannot be imposed in all its essentials on the past. Most scholars familiar with the historical arguments would probably agree with the measured summary of a medical historian, Vivian Nutton: 'If *Yersinia pestis* was the biological agent of the Black Death, as is still on balance the most likely explanation, its behaviour then, and for centuries afterwards, differed at times considerably from what has been observed over the last century and more. The symptoms of plague are recognizably the same, but its epidemiology and demographics are clearly distinct.'

The disease has changed its character with place and time, in other words—a conclusion wholly consistent with modern research. Not only do pathogens mutate, albeit much more slowly in the case of a bacillus like *Yersinia pestis* than in the case of viruses of various kinds, but other factors determining the epidemiology of plague vary even more markedly. The modern reservoirs of the disease include a great variety of rodents: rats in Madagascar and Vietnam, gerbils in Kazakhstan, meriones in Iran. Several species of flea can transmit it among rodents and then to humans, and some recent studies suggest that some of them may transmit it directly from one person to another. They have shown also that in Asia, Africa, and the Americas, plague is to be found in a variety of different climates and habitats. It affects different age groups in different parts of the world; and its human incidence and therefore its demographic outcome vary with standards of living and styles of housing, and with the behavioural responses of peoples and governments.

The most important recent contributions to our knowledge of plague, however, have come from the application of modern techniques of molecular biology to DNA recoverable from human archaeological remains in sites which can reasonably be associated with past epidemics. Since Nutton published his conclusions, several papers have appeared which make major and persuasive contributions. One of these papers, published in 2010 by an international group of scientists, used the technique of genome sequencing to trace the genealogy of *Yersinia pestis* found in its present locations. It concluded that the pathogen evolved in China or its vicinity more than 2,600 years ago, before producing different strains, or 'biovars', in different locations in the course of its subsequent evolution. Another paper, also in 2010, by a similar group, analysed evidence from seventy-six skeletons found in five possible plague sites in different European countries, all dating from the 14th to 17th centuries (see Figure 1). It found evidence of one or other of two different strains of the bacillus in all five sites, which suggested that the disease might have entered Europe by two different routes, and it concluded that this large body of evidence demonstrated 'unambiguously that *Yersinia pestis* caused the Black Death'.

That conclusion has been amply confirmed by similar work in recent years. It is becoming clearer also that the different strains of *Yersinia pestis* found in different places can be used as markers to trace the movement of plague across space as well as time. Part of the history of plague is recoverable from the archaeological and biological record of ancient DNA.

The historical record

More certain knowledge of the pathogen responsible and how it behaves tells us only a part of the history of past plagues, however. For most of the rest, historians have to rely on the written record, and that also has limitations which need to be recognized at the outset. The consistent use of the name plague for certain crowd diseases of severe form can often be supported by written descriptions of heavy mortality and distinctive symptoms, especially in the long sequence of European epidemics from the later Middle Ages onwards. Beginning with Michele da Piazza in the initial outbreak in Messina in 1347, chroniclers and physicians commented on buboes and other 'tokens' of plague like carbuncles, boils, pustules, and spots of various kinds, and used them along with the suddenness of death and the rapid transmission of the disease to distinguish it from other infections. An English chronicler was therefore able to separate cases of 'pestilence', plague, from cases of 'the pox', smallpox, when they coincided in an epidemic in 1369; and a few years later, a Florentine merchant made similar distinctions, stressing in his case the exceptional contagiousness of a disease which he and his contemporaries sometimes called simply 'the contagion'.

Nonetheless, there could never be absolute certainty about plague's identity. There were as many plague-deniers in the past as there have been more recently, often for good, if self-interested, reasons. The first reaction of many town authorities to an epidemic was to deny that it was plague until the evidence was plain for all to discern. To do otherwise was to provoke the flight of many of the citizens and disrupt local commerce, which is why 'slandering a town with plague' was a potent weapon for anyone disaffected. Doctors were subjected to similar pressures from patients and their families, given the social isolation that followed a plague diagnosis. Yet there was more than self-interest in the several cases of diseases being described as 'much like the plague but not the plague' or 'not the plague, but a disease somewhat akin to it'. It was the uncertainty of contemporary medical understanding that led Ambrose Paré, a 16th-century French physician, to reach the conclusion that because plague exhibited 'so great variety', it was 'very difficult to set down anything general or certain' about it.

One obstacle to understanding was the absence of any clear notion before the later 17th century that diseases were specific entities. Despite general agreement on plague's symptoms, it was thought possible for one disease to be transformed into another, so that 'spotted fever' (typhus) might turn from a 'plague-like fever' into the genuine article. The epidemiology of plague was as difficult to understand as its aetiology. Contemporary writers from 1348 onwards tried to grapple with questions such as why plague hit some countries or cities when others escaped. There was a variety of possible answers. At the individual level, doctors in the classical medical tradition going back to the Roman physician Galen looked to the constitution of the victim in order to discover what predisposed him or her to infection, and found the answer in an imbalance in the 'humours' whose equilibrium was vital to health. When it came to explaining infected localities, the Greek physician Hippocrates had directed attention to environments, to the weather and waters, and to the modes of housing and diet prevalent in particular places. And alongside all this, there was an equally long history to concepts of 'contagion' which explained how plague was transmitted from person to person, through breath or touch, or by exchange of clothes and property.

Although often embellished in different ways, these three approaches to disease, with their focus respectively on the individual, the environment, and modes of transmission, have been common to most cultures and civilizations susceptible to epidemics and crowd diseases. They have left ample room for argument about which of them had greatest importance, and in the case of European plagues, as we shall see later, there was often fierce controversy between those who attributed them to local environments and those who regarded contagion and transmission across space as fundamental. But the realities of epidemic situations meant that the three elements were usually combined in one mixture or other, and could reasonably be thought to have features in common. Notions of 'corruption' and 'putrefaction', for example, might be used to explain the imbalances in the humours which laid some individuals open to plague, and which also might account for the poisonous 'miasmas' in the air which spread plague in particular environments—and both kinds of pollution might cling to individuals and things and so contribute to the contagion which spread contamination, the smell of plague, from place to place.

Despite the uncertainties which gave some instability to definitions and interpretations of plague, however, most of the arguments in the past were about its nature, not about whether plague existed at all. They were part of prolonged and repeated discussions, between the 14th and 18th centuries, comparing the symptoms and modes of expression of a particular epidemic disease. In that period also, there were sources independent of the narratives of chroniclers and physicians which drove home the same message, and provided indisputable evidence of a particularly savage and rapidly lethal infection. In the 14th and 15th centuries, manorial records recording tenements left vacant testified to the impact of plague in rural areas, and from the 14th to 18th centuries, there were registers of wills, lists of deaths, and 'bills of mortality' in towns, all of them recording substantial increases in mortality for a few months in what other sources describe as years of plague (see Figure 12 in Chapter 4).

That was the historical reality of plague, and some of it was known to Europeans who encountered it later, when it had disappeared from Europe. They were able to observe it first, and almost immediately, in the Near East and North Africa in the later 18th and early 19th centuries. They then looked at it more closely in the Far East in the 1890s, and knew something about its presence earlier in 19th-century China. They had little doubt that what they saw on these occasions was the old 'bubonic plague' from which Europe had now somehow escaped, and that the bacillus they were searching for and ultimately isolated should be called *pestis*. Plague had a continuous history.

How far back that history extended before the 14th century was, and remains, much more uncertain. In the absence of independent evidence for the scale of epidemics, such as early registers of wills provide, much rests on the quality and quantity of the literary evidence alone. For the plagues of the 6th to 8th centuries, there are relatively full narratives of epidemics and descriptions of symptoms which clearly resemble those of the 14th century. They have left most historians in no doubt that the same disease was at work, and recent discoveries of ancient DNA confirm the identification. The same names—pestilence and plague—were applied to them in the Latin West, and there was a similar broad consistency in the terms used in the Syriac sources which describe them in other parts of the Mediterranean.

The evidence is much slighter for earlier epidemics, however. In the case of the most ancient plagues, like the 'plague of the Philistines' mentioned in the Old Testament or the 'plague of Athens' of 430 BC described by Thucydides, one can scarcely rest any retrospective diagnosis on the continuity of the name on its own; and modern attempts to identify the pathogens responsible, even where there is some archaeological evidence, have been wholly inconclusive. It must be doubtful whether such cases have a place in the *biological* history of plague, and a large question mark will hover over them in this book for that reason. They are part of plague's larger history, nonetheless, because the record that remains of them has had its own continuous existence over the centuries, and was brought into play and given fresh authority and resonance whenever the label plague was used.

In classical and Christian Europe, and in the Muslim Middle East, the Old Testament and Thucydides influenced the ways in which plague was interpreted and described. The Bible showed that sudden mortalities had supernatural causes and taught people to look for their origin in the workings of divine providence. Thucydides focused on how people reacted to them, and on the moral and social crises they caused. As we will see in later chapters, his description of wholesale flight from an infected city, left lawless, with corpses unburied, religious ceremonies abandoned, and physicians unable to find a cure, was a model for all later accounts of plagues—from Livy talking about an epidemic in Rome in 364 BC onwards.

It would be carrying scepticism to an extreme to say that literary conventions of this kind dictated what people saw, but they certainly taught people what to look for and record. There were few left alive to bury the dead, says Bede about a pestilence in 6th-century Britain, and a score of chronicles of 1348 echo him. 'Grass grew in the streets', says Paul the Deacon about Rome in a plague in 680, and Samuel Pepys about London a thousand years later in the plague of 1665. To a degree, interpretations and responses to plague were copied and taught, not reinvented and coined afresh whenever plague occurred. That may often have limited perceptions of the reality. But it was also part of a learning experience, especially when—as in Europe between the 14th and 18th centuries—plague epidemics were often repeated over a very long period. People learned how to avoid it, created ways of measuring and comparing one epidemic with another, and even developed mechanisms designed to mitigate its effects, as we shall see in Chapter 5. One of the continuities in the history of plague which justify this book was its educative function.

Framing histories of disease

It will be evident that historians of disease need to consider multiple facets of the phenomena they study. The social history of medicine as practised since the 1960s has been enormously fruitful in showing how diseases are in many respects 'social constructs'. It has drawn attention to the non-biological elements which shape their impact, all of which must have their place in later chapters of this book. They include the social and physical circumstances which govern their incidence and severity on any given occasion; the political and social attitudes and structures which determine public reactions to them; and the intellectual and cultural presuppositions which shape the ways in which they are interpreted. But historians must also pay attention to the biological phenomenon and the large part that biology plays in the complex interactions of environments, people, and pathogens that create epidemics.

Charles Rosenberg, one of the most penetrating of recent historians of medicine, points out that 'a disease does not exist as a social phenomenon until we agree that it does—until it is named'. But he goes on to insist that the names which distinguish a disease entity, and the modes of description and explanation which go with it, are not wholly arbitrary. The ways in which a disease can be defined are limited by its nature—whether acute or chronic, more or less easily transmitted between places and people, with high or low morbidity and mortality rates in the populations affected. Rosenberg therefore prefers the metaphor of a frame rather than a construct to denote how societies fashion their explanations and classifications of disease: 'Biology, significantly, often shapes the variety of choices available to societies in framing conceptual and institutional responses to disease; tuberculosis and cholera, for example, offer different pictures to frame for a society's would-be framers'.

The metaphor of picture and frame can profitably be applied to plague also. The portraits of plague painted over the centuries are visibly those of a distinctive disease: one with horrifying, painful, and recognizable symptoms; rapidly transmitted; and the cause of unparalleled personal suffering, social disruption, and communal discord. The ways in which the phenomenon was framed depended on the interests and intentions of the framers, however, and the particular colours, settings, and points of view they adopted changed over time.

Each of the following chapters has therefore been designed to introduce one of the frames into which plague has been set, either by contemporaries who reacted directly to the phenomenon or by later historians informed to a greater or lesser degree by the findings of modern medical science. Chapter 2 will introduce one of the frameworks which it has become conventional since the later 19th century for historians and epidemiologists alike to apply to the chronology of plague—grouping epidemics into larger 'pandemics', the first of them beginning in the 6th century. This frame gives some shape to plague's history, although it has a particularly artificial starting point around AD 540, as we shall see.

After 541, however, the record of plagues is sufficiently full to have persuaded many historians that *Yersinia pestis* was the pathogen involved. It is also sufficiently full to demonstrate considerable continuity, not only in the kinds of frame which have been applied to these epidemics, but in the common features which lie within all of them. Plague fully merits a single name and a single history.

Chapter 2
Pandemics and epidemics

The conventional picture of the history of plague divides it into three long pandemics, each of them made up of a series of separate but closely connected epidemics in particular places extending over centuries. The arrival of each pandemic was announced by a major epidemic explosion, hitting several cities and countries in rapid succession. There was then a tail, as it were, of plague outbreaks occurring at longer intervals and over smaller areas, until the disease apparently disappeared for a century or more before another pandemic erupted. That model (summarized in Box 1) is a retrospective reconstruction and it has its limitations, as we shall see. But it broadly fits with what the historical record tells us.

Box 1 Plague pandemics

FIRST: AD c.541–c.750 in Mediterranean and Europe

Initial major epidemics: the 'Plague of Justinian', 541–4

SECOND: 1347–c.1771 in Europe, c.1850 in Mediterranean

Initial major epidemics: the 'Black Death', 1347–52

THIRD: c.1894–?

Initial major epidemics: India, China, 1894–1922

Pandemics

The Greek historian Procopius described the initial eruption of the first pandemic as 'a pestilence by which the whole human race came near to being annihilated'. It had 'started from the Egyptians who dwell in Pelusium', a port at the eastern mouth of the Nile, and then spread to Alexandria in AD 541 and out across the whole of the Mediterranean. Procopius saw the severe mortality in Constantinople, and the Emperor Justinian himself contracted plague and recovered, hence the name given to that first great epidemic. Other contemporaries, writing in Latin and Syriac, and later chroniclers, using Arabic, refer to the plague in much the same terms, some (like Procopius) describing buboes, some saying the plague came to Pelusium from Ethiopia, all referring to its speedy transmission and heavy mortality. In the 540s, it reached as far as Persia and Ireland, and several waves of infection followed up to 750. There were two in England between 664 and 687, and the last one in the Mediterranean hit Naples in 747.

The sources for the second pandemic present a similar picture and are much more voluminous, partly because it lasted much longer. The course of the great initial wave, now known as the Black Death, can be mapped in some detail (see Figure 4). Plague came into the Black Sea, probably from the steppes of Asia, and then moved into the Mediterranean, where it hit Messina in Sicily in the autumn of 1347. By 1352, it had reached most of Europe, as well as North Africa and the Middle East, and it persisted there for centuries, with isolated incursions as far as Iceland by the 15th century and even perhaps some towns in Spanish Central America by the 16th. The last major epidemics in Europe were in the exposed port of Messina, once again in 1743, and in Moscow in 1771, but they continued on the southern and eastern shores of the Mediterranean, and in Asia Minor and the Balkans, into the 1840s.

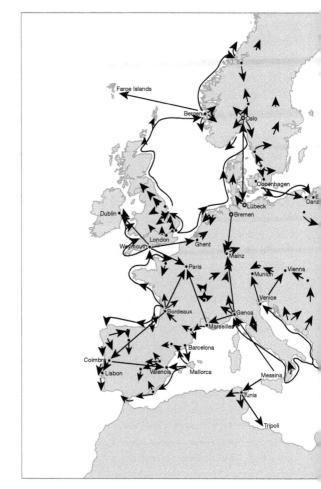

4. The spread of the Black Death, 1346–53.

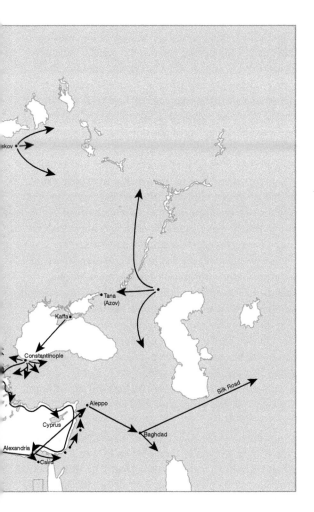

The arrival of a third pandemic was heralded by epidemics in Canton and Hong Kong in 1894. The disease had come from Yunnan, in south-west China, and once it reached ports at the hub of the Asian-Pacific trading network, it moved rapidly, causing major outbreaks in China, Manchuria, and especially India into the first decades of the 20th century, but having only a modest effect in other parts of the world. Minor outbreaks continue to the present day wherever animal reservoirs of the disease provide foci of infection, as in Africa, central Asia, and California, and it is likely that we are still in the tail of this third pandemic.

The initial epidemics of the third pandemic proved less serious than those of the first and second. Total deaths from plague in China and India between 1896 and 1910 have been put at around thirteen million—an enormous number. Given the size of the populations at risk, however, mortality rates were not as high as they had been during the Black Death, when there were an estimated twenty million plague deaths in Europe, and more than a third of the population probably died in five years. No one knows what the total mortality of the Plague of Justinian was, and there have been widely divergent estimates, but literary sources suggest that there may have been comparable depopulation in some parts of the Mediterranean world. The contrast between the heavy plague mortalities of the distant past and those of the 19th and 20th centuries is one reason why, as we saw in Chapter 1, some have doubted whether the disease responsible for the third pandemic can have been the same as that which caused the first two.

The pandemic model which is the topic of this chapter presents puzzles of its own, however. The most obvious feature of the picture presented in Box 1 is that it is one created by Western eyes, by people in Constantinople or Rome, Paris or London, looking at the parts of the world where they had commercial or imperial interests. The global history of plague might look very different if Chinese and Indian accounts of ancient epidemics, of which there are many, had been fully examined through modern medical spectacles; or if there were any records at all of similar outbreaks in sub-Saharan Africa before Europeans arrived. We cannot say what happened to plague before the first pandemic in Box 1, or between the first and the second, because we know next to nothing about the early history of epidemic disease in east Africa and central Asia, regions where plague has been endemic in modern times, and from one or other of which it probably moved north or west in AD 540–1 and 1346–7. Although it may have been the case, we cannot even be sure that in 540 plague came from central Africa rather than Asia, since contemporary references to Ethiopia may simply have been copied from what Thucydides had said about the much earlier Athenian 'plague' of 430 BC.

Plague is unlikely to have appeared from nowhere, *ex nihilo*, in AD 540, however. The Roman world of the early Christian era certainly knew of epidemics on the far side of the Mediterranean, in Libya, Egypt, and Syria, in the 3rd century AD and perhaps earlier, some of which may have been outbreaks of plague. It is even more improbable that plague disappeared altogether from the globe between the second and the third pandemic. In the early 19th century, it affected Malta and Noja, near Bari in southern Italy, between 1813 and 1815; and it was still prevalent until the 1840s in Egypt and the Ottoman Empire; and in parts of Russia until the 1870s. An outbreak of plague was reported near Bombay in India in 1836, and another in the Persian Gulf in 1876. Meanwhile, there had been a series of epidemics of uncertain character in Yunnan from the 1770s onwards, long before plague moved from there to Canton and Hong Kong to start the third pandemic in 1894. That may have been a fresh invasion of bubonic plague from its central Asian reservoir, but the second and third pandemics certainly overlapped chronologically.

The long interval from 750 to 1346, between the first and second pandemics, is much more difficult to fill. There are only stray references to what may have been plague in the Middle East in the 11th century, and none in the 12th or 13th. Chinese descriptions of epidemics over the same span of time are plentiful, but none has been persuasively identified as plague: at any rate, there are no clear references to buboes. Once again, however, plague must have been active somewhere, perhaps occasionally moving beyond the rodents in its usual reservoirs, even if it did not break out into human epidemics. But the gap between the early and late medieval pandemics in the West suggests that epidemic plague could and did disappear—not from the globe—but from vast areas, and notably from Europe between the 8th and 14th centuries and again after the 18th. The history of the first two pandemics also indicates that there was something wholly unusual about the Plague of Justinian and the Black Death, the two great explosions that inaugurated a succession of European plagues. There has been nothing quite like them in recorded history.

Appearance and disappearance

Despite its limitations, therefore, the pandemic model raises some important historical questions. Why was it that plague appeared in Europe with a bang then, in 541 and 1347, and not at some other time; and why did it disappear, less with a bang than a whimper, when it did? Sudden and dramatic as their arrival was, the initial causes of pandemics have attracted more attention than the reasons for their gradual and never wholly certain disappearance; and neither phenomenon can be attributed with any certainty to one single cause. The number of variables involved in the interactions between disease and the human and natural environments which shaped it means that there are several potential determinants of the outcomes, probably acting together, perhaps in random ways. The two questions have therefore been approached from a number of different angles. To use the metaphor employed in Chapter 1, they have been 'framed' from different points of view.

One influential approach, first fully elaborated by W. H. McNeill in his *Plagues and Peoples*, focused on the global exchange of infections over the centuries between widely dispersed 'pools' of disease. The introduction of 'new' diseases to crowded populations not yet adapted to them, generally through new avenues of trade, conquest, or colonization, disturbed local ecological balances between pathogens, parasites, and humans with lethal consequences. From that point of view, the first pandemic can be seen in general terms as the product of movements and interactions created by the Roman Empire and the early barbarian invasions of the West; and its starting point, the Plague of Justinian, might be ascribed more particularly to diplomatic and commercial contacts between Byzantium and both Ethiopia and Arabia around AD 500, which provided links with African or Asiatic sources of infection.

That might seem explanation sufficient for the purpose, but there is an alternative view. Hitherto stable patterns in the distribution of disease and prevalence of infection may have been disrupted, not by human movement, but by sudden changes in the climate. Studies of ice-cores and tree-rings (dendrochronology) have transformed our knowledge of past climatic fluctuations since McNeill wrote, and there is now hard evidence that a sharp deterioration in the weather coincided with the beginning of both the first and the second pandemic. Perhaps it was more than coincidence that a climatic shock, datable to the years between 536 and 545, preceded and accompanied the eruption of plague in 541. Precisely how the first fed through to the second remains to be established, however. Cooler and wetter climates may have brought more people more closely together, and hence increased the likelihood of infections being transmitted. Bad weather also caused poor harvests, and malnutrition might seem likely to have reduced human resistance to disease, but there appears to be no evidence that shortage of food increases vulnerability to bubonic plague. Alternatively, it might be that climate change had its most important impact, not on people, but on rodent populations in the

African and Asian reservoirs of plague. They cannot be left out of the discussion.

A third approach to the origin of pandemics has accordingly come from biological scientists interested in the ecology and demography of the mammals and their fleas which carried plague in central Asia in the second half of the 20th century and occasionally transmitted it to humans. Recent models of the dynamics of plague in its natural reservoirs there point to the ways in which wild rodent populations fluctuate, partly in response to changes in local climates. In Kazakhstan, the prevalence of plague among rodents (in this case gerbils) increases in warm springs and wet summers, when their populations grow and the risks of plague's transmission to humans within and beyond the initial reservoir multiply. Different species of rodent and flea react to different climatic conditions in different ways, which complicates an already complex picture. It has been suggested, however, that lower temperatures in the 530s expanded the rodent reservoirs of plague in central Africa, pushing their boundaries eastwards and thus linking them more closely with trade routes leading to Ethiopia and the Red Sea.

In the case of the first pandemic, therefore, it is possible to identify alternative initial causes, springing from shifts in human behaviour, the weather, or rodent ecology. We might call them potential triggers of the epidemic explosions that followed, and it may be that all of them interacted in intricate ways impossible to disentangle at this distance in time. Much the same can be said about the origin of the second pandemic, for which the historical evidence is fuller, and has been more closely analysed and vigorously debated. Here, however, recent work has focused particularly on climatic change, which has come to be understood as far more than the small trigger for an explosion that required other material to create it. It was in itself a hugely disruptive event with immediately disastrous consequences.

The tree-ring evidence leaves no doubt that there was unusually adverse weather across the northern hemisphere between 1314 and 1317, and again from 1343 to 1355. The first sequence of wet and cold summers caused famine throughout Europe between 1315 and 1322, and was followed by a highly contagious murrain of cattle, killing livestock all over the continent between 1316 and 1319. The second sequence, of course, accompanied the Black Death. As in the 540s, the links between weather and famine, on the one hand, and animal and human disease, on the other, may have been indirect, but the coincidences amply justify the conclusion reached by their leading historian, Bruce Campbell, that they amounted to a 'massive ecological dislocation' which led directly to a prolonged agrarian and demographic crisis in the early 14th century.

Previous historians of that European crisis had generally interpreted it in Malthusian terms, as the inevitable result of population pressing against available resources. In a Malthusian context, malnutrition and diseases of one kind or another were 'endogenous' events, necessary checks to further population growth, and if the Black Death had not served that purpose, something else, perhaps over a longer period, but sooner rather than later, would have had the same effect. Instead, Campbell forcefully argues, climate and disease need to be treated as independent 'exogenous' variables, and in this instance as 'historical prime movers to be analysed and understood in their own right'. The argument has been a salutary one, reasserting as it does the importance of the unpredictable in history and of environmental factors which can act as independent forces shaping events. But it also has its dangers. The search for prime movers and initial causes can be carried too far if it diverts attention from the phenomenon at issue—in our case, pandemics of human plague.

Historians are much more interested in what the historical evidence tells them happened further along the chain of events.

A model of good sense in this respect is Giovanni Boccaccio's non-committal account in his *Decameron* of what Florentines said about the Black Death in 1348:

> Some say that it descended upon the human race through the influence of the heavenly bodies, others that it was a punishment signifying God's righteous anger at our iniquitous way of life. But whatever its cause, it had originated some years earlier in the East, where it had claimed countless lives before it unhappily spread westward, growing in strength as it swept relentlessly on from one place to the next.

We might reasonably follow Boccaccio in looking to the East for the proximate origins of the Black Death, and turn away from climate for the moment and back to McNeill and the importance of human behaviour. McNeill pointed to the importance of the Mongol horsemen who laid siege to Kaffa in the Crimea in 1346, and probably carried plague with them from the Eurasian steppe to the Black Sea, giving it easy access to the Mediterranean. Alternatively, as one Florentine chronicler supposed, it is possible that it came by sea 'from China and upper India'. In either case, however, plague invaded Europe from outside, just as it had in the 6th century. These invasions were also exogenous events, as palpable as a climatic shock or a meteor strike. Yet they were themselves only a starting point. In order to have the impact that it did, plague also needed crowded cities linked by busy commerce to give it fuel and speed it on its way. It needed the historical processes of economic expansion and demographic growth which had occurred for a century and more before plague arrived in the 540s and 1340s.

The origins of the third pandemic—if it was a separate phenomenon—illustrate the same general point. So far as is known, there was no global climatic event to account for it, although local climates may have affected rodent population densities in western China in the ways suggested by modern studies of plague in central Asia. What seems more certain is that the first plague epidemics among humans were in Yunnan, where the development of mining in the later 18th century boosted populations, especially in towns, and where military campaigns during a Muslim rebellion between 1856 and 1873 provided ideal conditions for its transport further east. It depended as much on local conditions and human behaviour as on external impacts. Prolonged and devastating pandemics required a receptive context as well as initial causes.

It will be clear that historians have to contend with a plethora of potential and contested explanations for the origins of pandemics. When it comes to understanding their end, they face the opposite challenge of finding any persuasive explanation at all. No exogenous factors seem to explain the disappearance of plague from Europe in 750 and again in the later 18th century. There was no sudden alteration in the climate at the required points. The 'Little Ice Age', for example, did not prevent heavy plague mortality in London in the 17th century or Moscow in the 18th. With other infections, one might consider the possibility that long exposure to disease had conferred acquired immunity on human populations at risk, but there is no evidence that human plague infection produces natural immunity of that kind. It has been suggested that the withdrawal of plague in the middle of the 8th century might have been the result of the microorganism evolving in a way which gave rodents or even humans immunity to *Yersinia pestis*, but microbiologists now think that unlikely. The end of the first pandemic remains a puzzle, the greatest mystery in the whole history of plague.

The disappearance of plague from Europe in the 18th century may be easier to account for. Some possible explanations which have been suggested fail to convince. There is no evidence of plague declining in virulence or leaving resistant populations of humans or rodents behind it. Until their very end, European epidemics of plague were as lethal when they occurred as they had been in the later Middle Ages. They became increasingly restricted to major towns, but when they hit the same cities again and again, their severity hardly diminished over time. The last great plagues in Genoa and Naples in 1656–7 (see Figure 5) and Marseilles in 1720–1 carried off around half of the population; something approaching one-fifth of London's population in 1665; and one-third of Moscow's in 1771. The replacement of the black rat by the brown rat (a species much less inclined to nest close to humans), and improvements in hygiene and housing conditions which separated people from fleas and rodents even more effectively undoubtedly had an effect in the longer term. But there is little sign of it in the poorer quarters of west European towns as early as 1700 or in those in the east a century later. What remains is the possibility that deliberate human intervention succeeded in repelling the disease. A powerful case can be made that the quarantine precautions

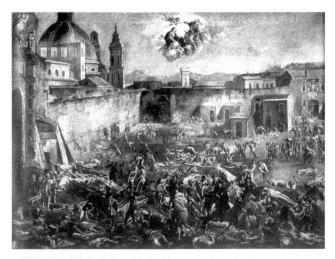

5. The Piazza Mercatello, Naples, in the plague of 1656, a contemporary painting by Micco Spadaro.

whose evolution will be described in Chapter 5 restricted the transmission of infection across long distances. They stopped plague in its tracks.

There were two prongs to European defences against plague in the early modern period. One was the isolation of ships coming from infected parts of the Mediterranean, the quarantining of their passengers, and the fumigation and sometimes destruction of their merchandise. Most of that apparatus, along with the monitoring of vessels and travellers by means of certificates of health, was fully in place in most west European countries by 1700. The second defence was a *cordon sanitaire* deliberately created between 1728 and 1770 in eastern Europe, along the heavily defended military frontier which protected the Austro-Hungarian from the Ottoman Empire. Patrolled by armed guards, and regularly reinforced whenever there was news of plague beyond the line, it similarly allowed suspect travellers, their goods, and even their cattle to be quarantined.

These practices were far from infallible, of course, not least because they were primarily designed to prevent the movement of human beings and their property, and only indirectly inhibited plague's transmission by fleas and infected rodents, who were the chief carriers of the disease. Quarantine of shipping did not protect Marseilles from plague in 1720, although a sanitary cordon around the city then stopped it moving much further into France. Chance undoubtedly played a part when precautions succeeded. Nonetheless, quarantine reduced the limits within which mere chance operated. It created protective thresholds which reduced the risk of plague retaining its hold across the whole European mainland. The map in Figure 6 shows the Austrian *cordon sanitaire* as it was in 1800, and also those areas (shaded) which continued to be reservoirs of plague—in the Balkans and Anatolia, as well as on the southern and eastern shores of the Mediterranean. Nothing could demonstrate more

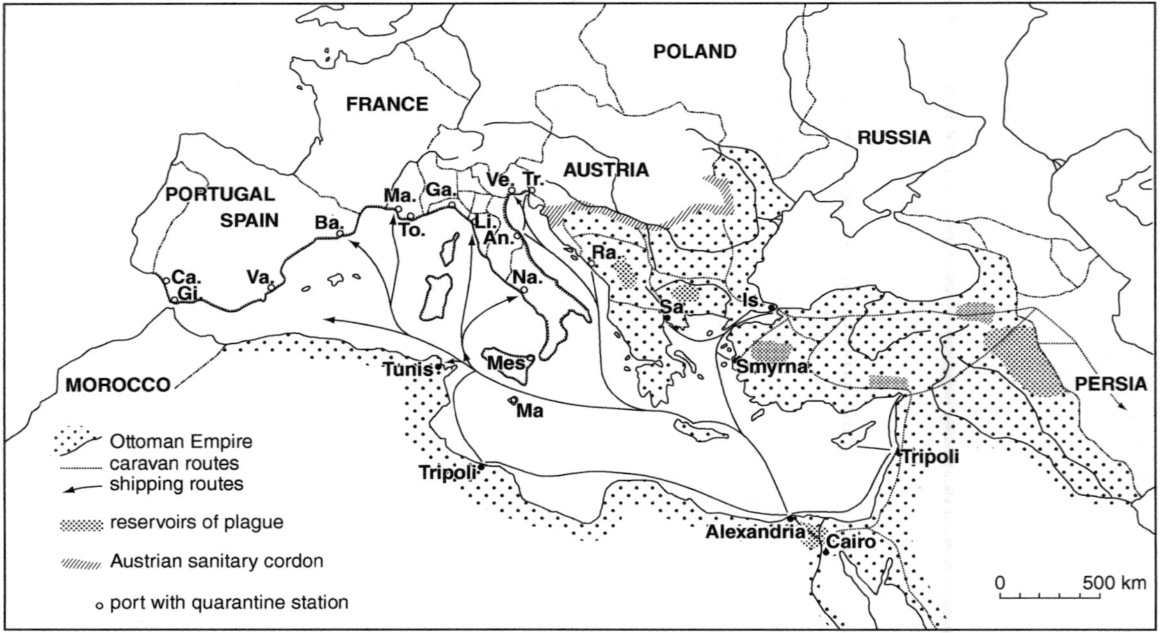
POLAND
FRANCE
RUSSIA
AUSTRIA
PORTUGAL
SPAIN
Ma.
Ga.
Ve.
Tr.
Ba.
To.
Li.
An.
Ra.
Ca.
Gi.
Va.
Na.
Sa.
Is.
Tunis
Mes
Smyrna
MOROCCO
PERSIA
Ma
Tripoli
Tripoli
Alexandria
Cairo
Ottoman Empire
caravan routes
shipping routes
reservoirs of plague
Austrian sanitary cordon
port with quarantine station
0
500 km

6. Plague in the Mediterranean, *c*.1790, showing the Austrian sanitary cordon and the areas of the Ottoman Empire (heavily shaded) where there were still reservoirs of plague.

clearly the *prima facie* case that this was what freed most of Europe from plague by the middle of the 18th century. Epidemics continued in the cities of the Ottoman Empire, like Cairo and Istanbul into the 1830s, when similar precautions to those taken in the West were being introduced and may help to account for the decline of plague there. It had left western Europe a century earlier.

In the 19th century, Britain and other countries initially relaxed their vigilance and modified their quarantine laws, and steamships rapidly carried plague back again in the early 20th century. Then, however, Europe was defended by improvements in public and private hygiene and the urban environment, and by the disappearance of the black rat. In Britain, cases of infection—in Liverpool, Glasgow, and Suffolk—were few and sporadic, and deaths from plague rarely exceeded a hundred anywhere in the West. Now, another century later, when we have antibiotics and other benefits of modern medicine, plague seems to be still more evidently under human control, even in parts of the developing world. That is not to say that it will remain so. The end of plague in Europe in 750 and its reappearance in 1347 stand as stark reminders of how much remains unknown and unpredictable about the behaviour of pathogens. But the historical record also suggests that deliberate and organized human action has a place among the many factors that govern the transmission of infection.

Epidemics

Much of what has been said about the beginning and ending of long pandemics can be applied to their component parts: the epidemics more constricted in time and space which hit smaller areas over a few years and caused severe mortality in towns and cities in a few months. They were exogenous in origin, coming in from outside, but then limited or aggravated by endogenous factors such as population density and living conditions, and by the ways in which people reacted to them.

One early account of how plague arrived and took hold in Marseilles in 588 vividly describes a typical sequence of events. According to Gregory of Tours:

> A ship from Spain put into port with the usual kind of cargo, unfortunately also with it the sources of this infection. Quite a few of the townsfolk purchased objects from the cargo and in less than no time a house in which eight people lived was completely deserted, all the inhabitants having caught the disease. The infection did not spread through the residential quarter immediately. Some time passed and then, like a wheat field set on fire, the entire town was suddenly ablaze with the pestilence.

That was a story often repeated and well documented throughout the second pandemic. Towards its end, plague came to Marseilles again in 1720; and the pandemic reached England in 1348 by sea, perhaps through Bristol or the small Dorset harbour of Melcombe (now part of Weymouth). The disease commonly hit one or two households first and then, after a short interval, spread rapidly, within and beyond the place first infected. It can be traced moving along established routes of travel, and it is no accident that ports like Messina and Marseilles, London and Naples feature again and again in even the briefest histories of plague. It moved along roads too, and had its most dramatic effects in cities, usually in the late summer and autumn, sometimes reviving again in the following spring. Yet there were many exceptions to this apparently orderly pattern. There were always towns along a road with only a few cases, and villages hard hit when their neighbours were spared. Even in the most serious outbreak, the Black Death itself, large areas of Central Europe seem to have escaped, and Milan did not have its first serious encounter with plague until 1361.

Sometimes wars and famines coincided with plague epidemics, and then increased exposure to infection, as they did in northern Italy in 1629–30 and in parts of France at the end of the 16th century. Sometimes plague preceded bad harvests, as in England in the 1590s, initiating a prolonged period of economic and social stress. The stresses were always greatest for the poor, and once the first great epidemics of the Black Death were over, plague had a visible and pronounced social concentration wherever living standards and overcrowding were worst. But its concentration among the poor was visible also because the rich had often left town and were no longer part of the population at risk. Flight was no guarantee of safety, however, since refugees sometimes carried plague with them, and quarantine procedures were scarcely infallible protection either. By the 17th century, they may have been sufficiently developed to have had some local effect. In England, for example, rapid action by municipal authorities to isolate the first infected households might sometimes prevent major outbreaks, as perhaps in Bristol in 1665, but similar activity failed in Norwich in 1665–6. On a larger scale, concerted action by groups of towns may explain why most cities in northern Italy were not hit hard by plague in 1656, when parts of the south and Naples were devastated by it, but even then Genoa was a notable northern exception.

The result was an epidemiological pattern as perplexing for contemporaries as it is frustrating for the historian who tries to describe it. One can understand why an astrologer in England during the Black Death thought only his arts could explain why plague

> affected some countries more than others, and why…it affected some cities and towns more than others, and why in one town it affected one street, and even one house, more than others, and why it affected nobles and gentry less than other people, and how long it will last.

Much more was involved in that than the disposition of the stars, but multiple determinants inevitably delivered unpredictable results.

One thing at least is clear. Once plague had been imported into Europe in 1347–8, it remained for centuries afterwards. It might invade individual countries and cities from outside, sometimes from the eastern Mediterranean, but it had established what has been termed an 'area-wide endemicity', just as it did in India and China during the third pandemic and probably in Europe during the first. The gaps between the epidemic waves which moved across the continent grew longer after the 14th century; and some cities evaded the disease for half a century or more, before they were visited again for a second or third time. But there was plague somewhere in Europe almost every year between 1348 and 1680, and it remained a major killer in the cities it affected into the 18th century. 'Plague comes seldom, but then very sore' was an English proverb current from the early 16th century, and learned by hard experience. Plague had become a familiar part of the landscape.

In late medieval and early modern Europe, plague was both an independent historical actor, coming from outside and altering, sometimes radically, the social and economic environment, and also a dependent variable, itself shaped by the environments it encountered and the ways in which people responded to it. Chapter 3 will try to explore that dichotomy further by looking at the occasion when plague appears to have had its greatest independent and long-term impact, the Black Death.

Chapter 3
Big impacts: the Black Death

It has often been supposed that major epidemic disasters must not only have extraordinary causes of the kind discussed in Chapter 2, but also produce extraordinary and wholly unpredictable consequences. The severity of their impact in the past seems fully to justify their incorporation into what might be called 'Great Disaster' interpretations of history, the contention that such crises changed the whole course of events, and that without them things would not have turned out as they did. It will already be evident that one purpose of this book is to draw attention to some of the limitations of such an approach to the complexities of historical causation. It leaves too much that is important out of account. It must be allowed, nonetheless, that there is something to be said for the Great Disaster argument in a limited number of instances. The arrival of smallpox in the Americas along with the Spanish conquistadors is one of them. Many factors determined the collapse of the Aztec and Inca Empires in the 16th century, but no historian would deny smallpox a decisive role in what happened, both in the short and the longer term. In some periods and places, plague had similarly disastrous potential.

This chapter will concentrate on the second pandemic in Europe, and focus especially on the Black Death which initiated it, because the case for big impacts is most easily established there. The third pandemic had less decisive long-term effects. Where its impact on mortality was worst, in parts of India and China in the decades around 1900, it did not transform the demographic and economic status quo. As we shall see in Chapter 5, it created panics and aroused cultural responses more extreme than other causes of mortality crises at the time, such as cholera and famine. But in other respects, it was simply one more affliction keeping mortality high and living standards low. It did not alter the biological and social environment in either the short or the longer term.

The Plague of Justinian, at the start of the first pandemic in the 6th century, may have had larger effects, immediate and sometimes lasting, though the evidence is scattered and difficult to interpret. There are signs of abrupt population decline in parts of Gaul and England, of land being suddenly plentiful and tenants difficult to find in Egypt, and of peasants moving from poorer to richer land in several parts of Europe. Yet these were local phenomena which may not have been replicated elsewhere. Large-scale arguments which have sometimes been advanced, to the effect that plague on its own weakened the military potential of Byzantium in the face of the armies of Persia and Islam, or that it caused the decline of the urban economies of the Roman Empire have therefore been difficult to substantiate. 'There was too much else going on', one historian comments, 'for the pandemic to be accorded a leading role' in such large historic events.

The Black Death (see Figure 7) presents a much more formidable test case for Great Disaster theories of history, however; and there is plentiful evidence which allows plague to be set alongside everything else that was going on, so that its independent role in the outcomes can be assessed. The first two waves of plague, between 1347 and 1352 and then in the years around 1360, cut the population of Europe by at least one-third, and it stayed low for a century afterwards. Labour became scarce and its price rose. In consequence, in much of western Europe the balance of power between employers and workers, and between landlords and tenants, shifted to the advantage of the latter, and so did the distribution of wealth. Old agrarian institutions like serfdom and villeinage declined when customary labour services could no longer be enforced, and the status and living standards of the majority of the population materially improved. Sectors of international trade catering for an elite market and the industries which supplied them were depressed, while internal trade and local industry grew to meet the demands of local markets. In the later 14th and early 15th centuries, old social and economic relationships broke down and were reconstituted in new and enduring forms.

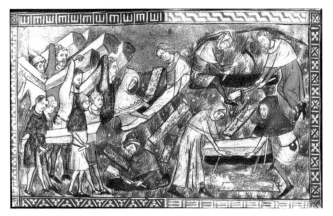

7. **Burying victims of plague in Tournai in 1349, the earliest surviving image of the immediate effects of the Black Death, from the annals of Gilles le Muisit.**

Other kinds of relationship, and the behaviour and attitudes of mind which underpinned them, may have been affected as profoundly. The initial shock of plague elicited extreme reactions like those common in other major disasters: a search for scapegoats—in this case the Jews, for example—and forms of religious enthusiasm intended to placate a hostile providence.

In the longer term, modes of piety and styles of artistic expression may have altered—both of them affected by shifts in patronage as wealth was redistributed and both perhaps responding to a new awareness of morbidity and mortality. There were many local variations in these outcomes, and none of them was wholly unprecedented. But plague in the later 14th century had an impact on every sphere of human activity, and it might well appear to have often been a prime mover, reshaping the course of European history.

Populations and economies

The case is strongest in the area where sudden, severe, and prolonged high mortality might be expected to have an impact—that of economic and social relations. The usual ties that bound farmers to their land, tenants to lords, and artisans and apprentices to their masters all became weaker when rents and the price of land fell, wages rose, and peasants, labourers, and even servants (female as well as male) had greater bargaining power and became more mobile. Matteo Villani was horrified by some of the consequences in Tuscany in 1363. 'Serving girls and unskilled women with no experience in service' now demanded high wages, while artisans asked for three times their usual pay, and farm labourers all wanted 'to work the best lands, and to abandon all others'. Consumer expectations rose alongside living standards:

> The common people, by reason of the abundance and superfluity that they found, would no longer work at their accustomed trades; they wanted the dearest and most delicate foods...while children and common women clad themselves in all the fair and costly garments of the illustrious who had died.

There were similar comments from an elite which felt threatened by rapid social change in England, where there is ample evidence of labourers moving to new lords and more fertile lands and of new employment opportunities opening up for women, and where the purchasing power of wages more than doubled between 1350 and 1450. The first of a series of ordinances trying to set a ceiling to high wages and prevent labour mobility in 1349 explicitly linked both phenomena to the death of 'a great part of the population, and especially workers and servants' in the recent pestilence; and in 1363, dismay at 'the outrageous and excessive apparel of many people, contrary to their estate and degree' prompted parliament to pass the first English sumptuary law, designed to regulate dress and diet according to social status. Ordinary labourers and artisans were scarcely wearing silks, but they could now afford better woollens than before, and the English textile industry grew in response to new consumer demand.

The case for regarding plague as the prime mover of economic and social change in the later Middle Ages thus has contemporary comment and much other evidence to support it. It nevertheless has some weaknesses. The most obvious arise from conspicuous differences between the consequences of plague in different places. Much depended on pre-existing economic conditions which determined whether demographic recession and labour mobility led to prolonged depression, or instead provided a stimulus to economic growth. Within England, for example, the less productive arable regions of the Midlands were less well placed to benefit from new opportunities than parts of East Anglia, and smaller towns were quicker to adopt new trades and employ immigrants than large cities, including London. Something similar lay behind contrasts on a larger scale. In Italy, Sicily recovered more quickly from 14th-century plagues than Tuscany, despite the fact that Sicilian plague mortality had been higher. In the Middle East, commercial and agricultural productivity declined more rapidly after the Black Death than in Europe, and failed to recover at all during the 15th century.

Pre-existing structures of power might also produce diverse outcomes. One of the starkest contrasts was between western Europe, where serfdom declined, and eastern Europe, where lords were powerful enough to impose it on previously free populations. The Black Death did not dictate the decline of serfdom, and in some circumstances, the institution disappeared without any help from plague at all. In Flanders, Holland, and much of Italy, it had already withered away in the course of the 12th and 13th centuries.

Ultimate outcomes depended finally on the duration of the demographic recession, and hence on the many factors which might explain why some populations recovered more quickly than others. The rise in popular living standards was particularly pronounced in England because its population did not begin to increase again until the early 16th century, and even in 1600 it was still lower than it had been in 1300. In France, by contrast, demographic recovery began much earlier (in the south from the 1420s), and populations in parts of the western Mediterranean had generally returned to their pre-Black-Death levels before 1550. It is no accident, therefore, that the first of many comments on the relative prosperity of the English as compared with the French peasantry, who ate no meat and only rye bread, comes from the 1470s. Similarly, when Italian visitors to England around 1500 thought the land uncultivated and its inhabitants lazy, they were reacting to the country's comparatively low population density. Contrasts of this kind were already separating some of the economies of north-western Europe from those of the south, despite shared experiences of plague.

It is not easy to explain why population remained low for long periods after the great epidemics of the later 14th century. Although recovery was quicker in some places than others, it was everywhere slower than Malthusian models would predict, given high wages and abundant cheap land. Mortality often remained high, especially in north-western Europe, where it may even have risen in the 15th century, elevated by diseases other than plague, whose outbreaks were more localized and generally less severe than before 1400. But fertility, which might have been expected to rise after mortality crises, also stayed low, and there has been much speculation about the possible reasons for that. In England, it has been suggested that the shortage of labour opened up employment opportunities for women and adolescents in trades and services, which delayed marriage and therefore the number of children born to each couple. Something similar may have been happening in parts of urbanized Tuscany, like Florence. There, it has been argued, the many people who enjoyed higher standards of living after the Black Death deliberately kept their fertility low, adjusting their decisions about marriage and family formation in order to maintain their new style of life.

In any event, it does not seem to have been plague, or at least plague on its own, which determined population trends in the 15th century, any more than it did in the 16th and 17th. At the end of the 16th century, despite continuing plague epidemics, European populations were rising again everywhere, and living standards for peasants and labourers, women as well as men, fell. The numbers of beggars and paupers increased, and there were famine conditions all over Europe in the 1590s. In the later 17th and early 18th centuries, populations were falling again, although plague was gradually disappearing from the continent altogether. They were depressed once again by rising mortality caused by other diseases and by changes in marital behaviour which affected fertility. After 1400, it would seem that plague never functioned as a lone historical actor in the great swings of demographic and economic fortunes across late medieval and early modern Europe.

If we are looking for explanations for long-term and large-scale economic and social change, therefore, it is impossible to attribute everything to plague. Too much else was involved in determining what were sometimes divergent outcomes. Yet this is not to suggest that the Black Death—an epidemic far more severe across the whole continent than any which followed—did not have a decisive effect in the short term. In parts of Europe, including England, populations had already been declining before 1348, and might have continued to do so if plague had not appeared, with results in the end similar to those which actually occurred. But the sudden and high mortality rates around 1350 greatly accelerated the pace of change, and in some places they may have initiated it.

In a searching analysis of the alternative models which have been employed to account for medieval economic change in England, John Hatcher and Mark Bailey conclude that none of them adequately explains why what occurred in the 14th century should have happened precisely when it did, and so quickly. Grand theories, based on Adam Smith, Marx, or Malthus, about commercialization, or the evolution of class relations, or the balance between population and resources are all found to be wanting, partly because they push plague too far into the background. Other factors determined the direction of historical change and its scale in any particular instance. Both depended on many things other than sickness and high mortality: on local circumstances and environments, and on the opportunities, inclinations, and relative power of different actors in the multitude of decisions which shaped economic and family relations. Nonetheless, the Black Death was responsible for the timing of change and the speed with which it occurred. In that sense, and in the short term, it was a prime mover of undeniable force.

Cultural turns

Precisely the same conclusion can be applied to historical changes that accompanied or followed the onset of plague in areas beyond the economic and the social, in the realm of ideas. The Black Death had a great deal to do with their timing, and much less with their character, which depended on local circumstances and what had gone before. Historians have assumed, with good reason, that epidemic shocks as severe as those of the later 14th century must have had an impact on how people thought about their world and their place in it, and some have argued that there were wholesale changes in mentalities, amounting to turning points in contemporary culture. Unfortunately, changes in habits of mind across whole societies are in the nature of the case more difficult to pin down than changes in the social structure, or the character and productivity of agriculture or industry. This is an area of historical inquiry where there has more often been rhetoric than scholarly precision, and yet it is one where being specific, as we shall see, pays dividends.

Some of the more extravagant assertions about the psychological impact of the Black Death need not detain us for long, therefore, although they have had a lasting influence. They originated with the first historical account of medieval plague across Europe, written by the German medical historian J. F. C. Hecker in 1832, at a time when cholera seemed about to recreate the horrors of the past. According to him, 'the mental shock sustained by all nations during the prevalence of the Black Plague' was 'without parallel and beyond description'. It destroyed confidence in the future; undermined deference and conventional moral norms; produced extremes of religious enthusiasm, and social and religious dissidence; and turned everything upside down. In effect, Hecker was building on late-medieval interpretations of the great pestilence as an apocalyptic catastrophe; and he created what has been well described as a 'Gothic' interpretation of plague which continues to colour many depictions of the later Middle Ages. Writing in 1893 about the Black Death in England, Cardinal Gasquet caught some of Hecker's tone. 'The Black Death inflicted what can only be called a wound deep in the social body, and produced nothing less than a revolution of feeling and practice, especially of religious feeling and practice.' It was 'a turning point in the national life' and 'the real close of the medieval period and the beginning of our modern age'.

Such grandiose statements have a place among the enduring images of plague considered in Chapter 6, and they have helped to sustain popular interest in the topic as well as stimulating argument among historians. Whether one conceives of the later Middle Ages as an era of darkness, obsessed with sin and fears of death, or as one of intellectual renaissance and incipient enlightenment, however, probably depends on personal predilection, since a case can be made for either. Plagues, like other natural disasters, challenge established ways of thinking, and may prompt intellectual innovation as well as doubt and dismay, but that trite observation scarcely takes us very far. The extent of plague's impact on mentalities is better measured by taking a narrower view and focusing on parts of the historical terrain where sudden mortality can be shown to have had a tangible effect.

Fourteenth-century changes of fashion in architecture and art have provided fertile territory from this point of view. Here plague had an immediate impact, directly by depleting the ranks of skilled artists and craftsmen, indirectly by reducing the incomes of cultured patrons among the elite and increasing those of people less able, and perhaps less inclined, to fund expensive artistic innovation. The triumph of the 'Perpendicular' style in English church architecture is an instructive case. Cheaper, because less labour-intensive, than its 'Decorated' predecessor, it took hold from the 1350s and was the architectural orthodoxy for the next 200 years. It might have caught on anyway, with or without plague, since there are earlier examples of it, as in the south transept of Gloucester Cathedral, which was finished by 1337, and probably in the cloister of old St Paul's in London, begun in 1332. But the consequences of the Black Death speeded the transition. It brought to a sudden close the great boom in cathedral and monastic building, which had been funded by the soaring agricultural profits of major ecclesiastical institutions in the 12th and 13th centuries. In its place, there was a proliferation of church building on a less lavish scale, paid for by local communities. No fewer than three-quarters of the surviving medieval churches of

England were built or rebuilt between 1350 and 1540, and in Perpendicular style.

Architectural fashions have less to tell us about modes of thought and feeling than other kinds of artistic expression, however. A classic study of painting in Florence and Siena in the 14th century takes us closer to mentalities, and into more controversial territory. In 1951, Millard Meiss claimed that there was a profound change of style and taste after the Black Death. There was a reaction against the humanistic innovations of Duccio and Giotto, and a return to less naturalistic and more austere styles, redolent of a simpler spirituality and more suited to an era dominated by plague: 'a darker realm of fearful, strenuous yet often uncertain piety, brightened only by mystical transports and visions of supernatural splendour'. There is more than a hint of Gothic extravagance in that argument, and it has often been disputed. Some of the works fundamental to Meiss's case, including the frescoes depicting the 'Triumph of Death' in the Camposanto at Pisa, probably pre-date the plague, for example. At the same time, it may well be the case that there was a reversion to more traditional styles when an enlightened elite of rich patrons, like the ecclesiastical authorities of Siena, were no longer able to afford the grandiose and innovative works they had funded in the past. The vast extension to the cathedral at Siena, begun in 1348, remains unfinished, a stark reminder of what a single munificent sponsor had once been able to contemplate.

What seems certain, however, is that Meiss's 'darker realm' was not all-pervasive. If we place artistic and architectural endeavours in their proper context, alongside other forms of pious and charitable investment, we find novelty as well as conservatism. In England, the quality of manuscript illumination, wall paintings, and even monumental brasses may have declined after 1350, but there were alternative and large collective investments in much more than Perpendicular churches. New foundations after 1348 included scores of chantries, new colleges at Oxford and

Cambridge, and new funds to support the poor, now deliberately targeted at the most 'deserving' (not wandering beggars and vagrants). Many of these were designed primarily to provide prayers for the souls of the benefactors, and surviving wills display a similar concern with death and the afterlife. But alms and almshouses and university colleges also provided benefits for the living, and so did the many fraternities paid for by local subscriptions which by the 15th century sustained sociability and mutual aid in English parishes.

Lay piety turned in similar directions elsewhere in western Europe after the plague. In Italy, testamentary bequests tended to focus on the family, often providing for memorials as well as prayers for the dead, but they also included bequests for dowries for girls from the deserving poor, and for the foundlings and orphans whose number multiplied in plague-time. The first European hospital exclusively for orphans was founded in Paris in 1363, and there was another in Florence early in the next century. There is no sign here of the breakdown of family ties and neighbourhood loyalties lamented by some of the contemporary chroniclers of epidemics. Neither can it be seen in the literature of the later 14th century, which included a remarkable group of Welsh poems expressing grief at the death of children during plagues. Rather, there is an evident concern to preserve the memory of the dead and equally to provide for the most vulnerable of those who survived.

Much of this evidence from testamentary and literary sources would support the view that plague helped to give death a more prominent place in popular mentalities. Such a shift of perception is suggested by the new forms of artistic and literary expression which have been used by many historians to demonstrate the pervasive appeal of macabre themes in the later Middle Ages. Although they mostly come from the 15th century and not the later 14th, and often from northern and not southern Europe, they

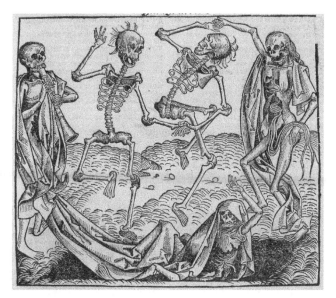

8. A Dance of Death from the late 15th century.

illustrate a world with very different ways of thinking and feeling from our own. One example is the image of the 'Dance of Death', the *danse macabre* (see Figure 8). Its earliest known representation was on a mural in the cemetery of the Innocents in Paris, painted in 1424–5, and it was for centuries afterwards an iconic representation of the inevitability and unpredictability of mortality, striking rich and poor, virtuous and vicious alike. The same message was driven home by the *transi* tombs of bishops and other notables, showing their corpses in various stages of decomposition, and by books on the *ars moriendi*, 'the art of dying well', illustrated with exemplary death-bed scenes, which had earlier antecedents but flourished after 1408 and taught the literate how to prepare for their end. Some of these images seem grotesque to modern sensibilities in societies in which dying has become a more private affair, but in the context of their time, they are fully intelligible. They were ways of confronting realities, including the deaths of thousands in plague-time, and making them, to some degree, comprehensible.

The same might be said about two more dramatic phenomena, much more closely tied to the Black Death itself, which Hecker emphasized and which a great deal has been made of since: the pogroms inflicted on Jews, who were accused of spreading plague by poisoning wells and rivers; and the punishments which crowds of penitents, 'flagellants', inflicted on themselves (see Figure 9). Both of them prominent in 1348 and 1349, and both of them the result of apocalyptic interpretations of the Black Death as a sign that the Last Days of the world were at hand, they have sometimes been cited as instances of collective and almost psycho-pathological hysteria in critical circumstances. The pogroms were undeniably rapid and popular responses to rumours and scares, and horrific in their violence. Nearly a thousand of Strasbourg's Jews were burned on an island in the Rhine in 1349, and the large Jewish communities elsewhere in the Rhineland were almost wholly exterminated.

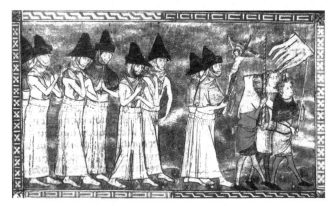

9. A procession of flagellants in 1349.

Yet these were massacres with some precedents behind them in the 1320s, and they were generally undertaken by due legal processes sanctioned by local authorities. Once magistrates began to have doubts about the evidence, and that came very quickly, persecution stopped. There were no more instances after 1352, except in 1360 in parts of Poland, which had scarcely been affected by plague earlier. There were to be similar scares about people deliberately spreading plague in later epidemics, but they were less widespread, easily restrained by judicial processes, and they scarcely amount to evidence of a mass hysteria typical of plague-time.

The flagellant processions were as common as persecution of the Jews immediately after 1348, and they continued into the early 15th century. Marching along the roads across much of Europe proclaiming the need for repentance in the face of God's evident judgements, their participants scourged themselves as they went, 'wearing hoods and beating themselves with whips until the blood flowed' according to a chronicle from Tournai. There had been similar movements earlier, one as early as 1260, but such autonomous expressions of religious enthusiasm without obvious official sanction in 1349–50 horrified ecclesiastical authorities. After that, the Church took them on board and exercised more control. When plague threatened Florence in 1399, there were more respectable processions of the 'Bianchi', who walked through the city and suburbs barefoot and dressed in white. One of the penitents participating was the great commercial tycoon Francesco Datini, the merchant of Prato, and his description of the occasion gives the impression, as his modern biographer remarks, of 'a gigantic nine-days' picnic'. There is no sign there of the hysteria there might possibly have been forty years earlier. It was a popular and pious outlet for stress, but it had become a wholly respectable affair.

These instances suggest that there was little that was wholly instinctive or irrational in popular responses to plague after

1348–9. Once the initial, apocalyptic shock of the Black Death had been absorbed and the challenges presented by epidemics become familiar, people adjusted their behaviour and adapted their ways of thinking so that they could accept them—not as something commonplace or everyday, but as inescapable facts of life. Plague was being accommodated.

Accommodating plague

Accommodating plague took less time than one might imagine. Parts of the process can be seen, once one looks for them, even in the first epidemics of 1348. In Marseilles, for example, where there was exceptionally high mortality in the first quarter of that year, local institutions proved flexible enough to cope with the consequences from the start. Local courts handled a flood of business, as heirs and claimants to vacant fields, houses, and bequests presented their cases; and they facilitated the upward social mobility of modest men and women by registering the sales and leases of property they could now afford. The town council responded to changes in the labour market by setting the wages of workers in fields and vineyards at levels much higher than before the epidemic. There was much more activity in the marriage market too, as widows or widowers remarried and newcomers to town found partners and started families. The number of weddings rose to two or three times its pre-plague level. One historian of the Black Death in Marseilles concludes that the social and institutional fabric of the town held together and proved 'remarkably adaptive'. It was an adaptability 'characteristic of a society that was both open and flexible, not the rigid and brittle affair imagined by Cardinal Gasquet and others' who depicted society's total disarray and dissolution in 1348.

Interpretations and perceptions accommodated the phenomenon as effectively as social institutions and practices, if not immediately in 1348, certainly over a very short period.

Chroniclers of the first wave of plague commonly noted, as Thucydides had done of the plague of Athens, that physicians had no remedy for it; and they found the causes of plague in unusual weather events, in the stars, and in the justified punishments of God. Physicians themselves initially agreed, among them the authors of the first of the 200 or so European plague tractates which survive from the century following 1348. An influential report from the Medical Faculty of Paris in 1348 became a model for others, beginning its account of causation with an unfavourable conjunction of Jupiter, Saturn, and Mars which had occurred in 1345. Samuel Cohn, the historian who has given these sources closest attention, notes, however, that there was a 'change in mentality' almost immediately after the Black Death. 'After 1350, we hear no more of the floods of snakes and toads, black snows that melted mountains, or the presage of earthquakes, and little of astrology or even God.' When plague returned in the 1360s, some chroniclers and medical writers began describing epidemics in more detail, pointing to regularities in their incidence, and drawing more optimistic conclusions.

Physicians now claimed, no doubt with considerable wishful thinking, that the therapies they advocated, including blood-letting and various ointments, had been shown by 'experience' to be effective. By 1415, Giovanni Morelli was able to reflect on six recent waves of plague in Florence, and assert that 'even if disasters still occur, I truly believe that some remedies work'. Experience of the social circumstances which brought or aggravated epidemics also taught other, perhaps more persuasive, lessons. Divine providence was still acknowledged to be the first cause of plague, but its secondary causes, more immediate and observable, were given increasing attention. There was as yet no general agreement, as there was to be from the 16th century onwards, that the poor were commonly the main victims: opinion about the social incidence of plague was divided. But opinion was unanimous about the aggravating effects of overcrowding and poor hygiene, and chroniclers of Pistoia in 1362 and Padua in 1405, and the Medical

Faculty of Prague in 1411, all noted plague's association with wars and famines.

Medical writers were also emphasizing another, more obvious lesson from experience: that plague was communicated by 'infection' through various means, including person-to-person contact. Members of the English parliament noted in 1439 that the disease was 'most infective' and that those infected by it should be avoided, citing 'noble physicians and wise philactradephers' as well as 'experience' in their support. There was a growing conviction that plague was gradually being understood, that attention to personal cleanliness and public sanitation might pay dividends, and that mere fatalism should be avoided at all costs. The very thought of plague and death might itself cause infection, many plague tracts insisted. Self-confidence was essential.

Overall therefore, changes in mentalities and social and economic behaviour do not leave the impression of a society passively suffering from an apocalyptic disaster which shattered existing institutions and ways of thinking and doing things. Rather, they show people coming to terms with a new kind of world, while employing many of the structures and frames of mind of the old. In a striking phrase, Cohn remarks that after 1348 plague was 'rapidly becoming domesticated'. Accommodating plague involved people making their own histories much as they had always done. They found ways of coping with disease and death, combating their effects, and creating explanations and images which, however inadequately, helped people to understand them. Those are the themes to be explored in Chapters 4–6.

Chapter 4
Private horrors

Recreating the private experience of plague-time, what it felt like to be in an infected town, is not as easy as might be thought. It is not simply that there is little direct testimony from the illiterate who suffered most, which is often the historian's problem. The difficulty lies also in the repetitive nature of the narrative sources which we have to use in its place. The shadow of Thucydides and the plague of Athens fell across most writers who tried to describe later plagues. Whether they had read Thucydides for themselves or drew on other chroniclers and authors who had, they inherited a narrative framework and illustrative images they felt bound to copy.

Like Thucydides, some of them would have said that they wanted 'merely to describe what it was like' in a plague, but they were equally tempted to exaggerate for dramatic effect, and equally determined to produce a story with a moral, about the collapse of all civil and civic standards of behaviour. They emulated his description of a 'catastrophe...so overwhelming that men, not knowing what would happen to them, became indifferent to every rule of religion or law', abandoning funeral ceremonies and respect for the dead, seeking only 'the pleasure of the moment' in 'a state of unprecedented lawlessness'.

None of this was total invention, and not all the motifs Thucydides inaugurated were exaggerations. People were in reality 'dying like flies' and being 'afraid to visit the sick', for example, and bodies were 'heaped one on the top of the other' and 'lying about unburied'. Thucydides caught the infection himself and had good reason to think 'the sufferings of individuals' were 'almost beyond the capacity of human nature to endure'. But it is difficult to separate reality from rhetoric in many of the later crafted narratives which were governed by precedents and expectations. One purpose of this chapter is to look beneath and beyond them, partly by noting topics which they included and Thucydides did not, partly by searching for alternative testimonies.

For the first pandemic, beginning with the Plague of Justinian, narrative sources are almost the only evidence we have. They tell us about whole households dying when plague took away masters as well as servants, streets made impassable by piles of stinking corpses, and 'all the customary rites of burial' abandoned. In Constantinople, bodies were buried in a common burial ground, then in extra pits hurriedly dug, then heaped up along the shoreline. John of Ephesus visualized plague as a wine-press, the 'wine-press of the fury of the wrath of God', and observed its victims thrown into pits and literally 'pressed down...trampled down like spoilt grapes' in order to make room for more.

Not all was dissolution and dismay, however. Many of the chroniclers were churchmen, and religious institutions and practices appear to have retained much of their hold. Only a handful of instances of newly converted Christians reverting to paganism were reported during epidemics, though that occurred in Paris and parts of the Middle East in the 6th century, and in Essex when plague first hit Britain in the 7th. As a general rule, the Christian Church seems to have proved more powerful than the oracles and temples of the Athenians, and the reassurances its ceremonies offered more popular than some clerical writers of the time would have us believe. Sermons were still being preached and listened to, and those that survive in manuscript form tell us what people who heard or read them were told to think about.

They were taught that plague had a supernatural origin, and generally interpreted it as a divine punishment for their sins. It could only be prevented or averted by public repentance and prayer, and without them no other remedies could have any effect. Lessons about the kinds of behaviour which were appropriate in plague-time followed from that, and contemporary references to them show that literate people at least were aware of the demands they made.

The most fraught issue was that of flight. Disagreements about its legitimacy were common in later centuries, and already being voiced in the 6th century. 'Flee fast, far and for a long time' was advice often repeated on the authority of the Roman physician Galen, and a survival strategy no less often qualified, and sometimes totally condemned, by ecclesiastical writers. In 726, Pope Gregory II roundly declared that flight was always 'the height of folly, for no one can escape the hand of God'. Some Calvinists were still taking the same hard predestinarian line in 1600, but by then many writers, clergy as well as laymen, had found a middle ground. Flight might be allowed, but not for those with weighty moral obligations, for heads of households, for example, who must attend to sick relations (unless they were confident that there was other support), and for magistrates and clergy whose obligations extended to the whole community of a city or a parish. In effect, the decision was left to individual consciences.

Whatever their obligations, there were always many people who fled, though not without qualms about doing so, as we shall see. Many others, including the poor, had nowhere to flee to. Paul the Deacon plainly exaggerated when he reported that after plague hit Liguria in 565, 'all had departed and everything was in utter silence. Sons fled, leaving the corpses of their parents unburied;

parents forgetful of their duty abandoned their children.'
Gregory the Great, elected Pope Gregory I in 590 when plague
killed his predecessor, described the many houses left empty in
Rome but also the grief of parents who stayed, going to the
funerals of their children and seeing 'their heirs march before
them to the grave'.

For those who remained to face the epidemic, Gregory organized
processions to demonstrate collective penance, one of them
(see Figure 10) later pictured with the pope himself leading it,
and raising his arms in supplication to St Michael the Archangel,
who is shown sheathing his destructive sword in response. That
apparently effective defence against plague is still commemorated
in the statue of St Michael on the Castel Sant' Angelo, which is
one of the two enduring images of plague with origins in the first
pandemic. The other is the figure of St Sebastian (see Figure 11),
always depicted riddled with arrows, which evoked the pains of
plague and referred back to God's arrows of destruction in the
Psalms of David, and to the arrows of Apollo, 'god of plague', in
Homer's *Iliad*. Prayers were said to him in plague-time from at
least 680 onwards (see Figure 11).

The plague of Justinian has left little lasting evidence about other
kinds of behaviour which might tell us something about how
people coped. Some cities had public physicians, apparently in
great demand during epidemics, but we know nothing about what
they offered their patients. One or two authors had lived through
more than one plague, like Evagrius Scholasticus writing in
Antioch, who had seen four since 542, when he had swellings and
fevers himself as a boy of 6. In the later epidemics, he lost servants
and relations, including a wife, daughter, and grandson, but he
tells us no more. More immediately poignant, and evocative of the
personal stresses of plague, even if they were invented, are reports
that people in Constantinople and Alexandria would only leave
home if they had written tags round their arms or necks giving
names and addresses, so that relatives could come and get them in

10. Pope Gregory the Great leading a procession during the plague of 590 in Rome, from a 15th-century manuscript.

case of sudden death. Such fragments show that there were survivors as well as victims, but little about how many of them there were, and how they coped in the face of catastrophes which posed daily predicaments. The historical records of the second pandemic help us to fill some of the gaps.

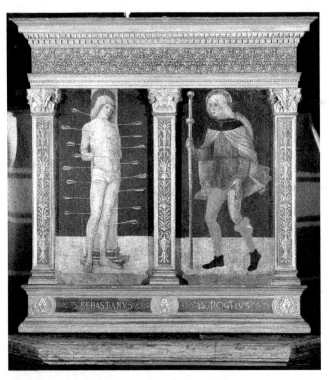

11. Plague saints, Sebastian and Roch, pictured in 1475.

The toll of death

Much of Boccaccio's eye-witness account of the Black Death in
Florence in 1348 echoes those of the past. 'All respect for the laws
of God and man had virtually broken down.' Funeral ceremonies
were neglected, and people took to drink and 'behaved as though
their days were numbered'. Bodies were carried off on planks,
because formal funeral biers were in short supply, and piled up in
specially dug trenches. The smell of rotting corpses was all
around. 'What more remains to be said?', he asked, in conclusion;
and he found something wholly novel—numbers.

It was 'reliably thought that over a hundred thousand human lives were extinguished within the walls of Florence'. The figure was too large, since modern research suggests that 50,000 or so may have died, perhaps 60 per cent of the city's population—but the dead were now being counted.

For our own estimates of mortality in the plagues of the 14th and 15th centuries, we have generally to rely on modern calculations of the size of a town like Florence before and after an epidemic, or on partial evidence from registers of wills and lists of deaths in religious institutions compiled at the time. Where such research has been undertaken for other cities during the Black Death of 1348–52, it suggests similar proportions. Plague probably killed nearly half the population of Siena, for example, and much the same percentage in London, Norwich, and Bury St Edmunds in England. From the 15th century onwards, such calculations can be more securely based on registers of deaths in parishes and on 'necrologies' or 'bills of mortality', which sometimes cover whole cities and in a few cases distinguish deaths caused by plague from those attributed to other causes. The quality of these sources varies, and in general they are fuller for epidemics at the end of the pandemic than at the beginning. By the end of the 17th century, however, we can begin to arrive at some round numbers which probably provide realistic estimates of total deaths and death rates in infected cities.

In the last major plagues in Italy, for example, something like 150,000 people (perhaps half the population) died in Naples in 1656–7; 60,000 (nearly 60 per cent) in Genoa in the same year; 28,000 (more than 60 per cent) in Messina in 1743; and that takes no account of rural plague mortality, which was particularly severe in Italy. During the last great plague in England in 1665–6, just under 20 per cent of Londoners perished (97,000 burials), but nearly half the people in Colchester (5,000). Mortality in the last great French epidemic, in Marseilles in 1720–1, also reached 50 per cent (50,000 deaths). Moscow's final great plague in 1771 killed 52,000, an estimated 20 per cent of the population. One can pile up numbers and proportions during epidemics in European cities like bodies in a plague pit; and the numbers were equally large, although the proportions were generally smaller, in some of the later plagues in great cities in the Middle East: 100,000 (20 per cent of the population) in Istanbul in 1778, for instance; and 60,000 (also 20 per cent) in Cairo in 1791.

Nothing like that was to occur in large cities in a single year during the third pandemic, not even in Bombay, where one of the worst plagues, in 1903, killed tens of thousands but only 3 per cent of an urban population of 800,000. What was special about the second plague pandemic was its capacity to create huge mortalities in crowded cities for centuries, even when it had lost the virulence in rural areas and scattered hamlets which was so remarkable during the Black Death. In great towns until the 18th century, plague had the potential to recreate the havoc which Boccaccio and Thucydides had described.

Plague epidemics had other features which make mere numbers of casualties and proportions of populations inadequate summaries of their horrors. Registers of wills and bills of mortality show that most of the deaths occurred in less than a year (see Figure 12), often in no more than three months, usually in the summer and autumn in Europe, although that depended on climate and the time of year that the disease arrived. The worst months were June to September in northern Italian cities in 1348, but December 1348 to May 1349 in London, where plague arrived later. In 1665, the disease reached London in April, and August to October were the cruellest months, when 60,000 deaths were attributed to plague.

Turning numbers of casualties into proportions of pre-plague populations, moreover, takes no account of flight, the hundreds, even thousands, who left cities if they could afford it and were free to do so. Mortality rates among the population actually at

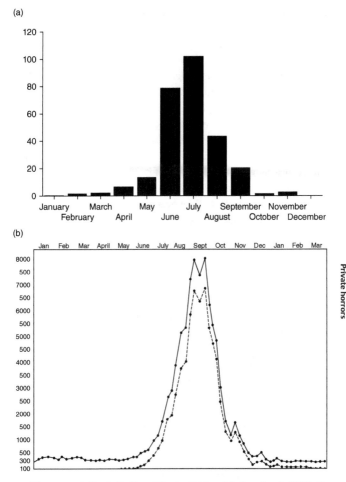

120

100

80

60

40

20

0

January   March   May   July   September   November
    February   April   June   August   October   December

(b)

Jan   Feb   Mar   April   May   June   July   Aug   Sept   Oct   Nov   Dec   Jan   Feb   Mar

Private horrors

8000
500
7000
500
6000
500
5000
500
4000
500
3000
500
2000
500
1000
500
300
100

12. **Plague mortality in Italian cities in 1348 and in London in 1665–6:**
(a) numbers of wills registered monthly in 1348 in Arezzo, Assisi,
Florence, Perugia, Pisa, and Siena; (b) weekly burials in London in
1665–6 (the dotted line indicates those attributed to plague).

risk must generally have been larger than the percentages already cited, except where the erection of sanitary cordons effectively limited flight, as perhaps from Marseilles in 1720–1. In order to gauge the full impact of plague, we need finally to take account of those who caught the disease and subsequently recovered. We know nothing about case-fatality rates attributable to bubonic plague in the distant past, but in modern times they ranged between 40 per cent and 60 per cent. It is possible therefore that relatively low mortality rates often conceal very high morbidity rates, and that twice as many people sometimes caught plague as died of it. The numbers and proportions suggested by historians, eloquent as they are, are more likely to understate than overstate the ravages of plague during the second pandemic.

The numbers nevertheless reinforce the impression given by literary sources that plague-stricken cities were environments dominated by death. When the number dying was at its height, there must have been many which looked like the Naples painted by Micco Spadaro in 1656, with corpses heaped up or buried haphazardly in pits, in squares, or outside city walls (see Figure 5). Keeping complete and accurate record of them was an impossible task, though many parish officers tried. In the middle of a London epidemic in 1563, one parish clerk was reduced to registering the burial of 'two corpses' or 'three corpses' without further identification. Another clerk, in 1625, sometimes found 'twenty or thirty corpses left at the place of burial' without any indication of their identity. In smaller places, parish registers could be more informative, and some had poignant stories to tell. The parish clerk of a Cheshire village in 1625 recorded that plague was brought in by Ralph Dawson, coming home from London, and infected his whole household. Ralph and a servant died first, and then a brother who died in a ditch. Ralph's uncle, close to death and too heavy for the survivors to carry, dug his own grave and lay down in it 'and so departed out of this world'.

The formalities surrounding death and burial were nevertheless maintained wherever possible, even if truncated, and even in great cities. The Black Death in Cairo killed more than 200,000 people between September and December 1348, over one-third of the population. Once again, there were not enough coffins to go round, although they were manufactured in great quantity and in haste. Bodies were carried on planks and camels to open trenches. According to contemporary accounts, the streets were full of mourners crying and wailing, as was traditional in Muslim funerals. The noisy equivalent in Christian cities was the tolling of church bells, knells announcing funerals and passing bells indicating that someone was close to death, incessant reminders 'of our mortality', as one Londoner remarked in 1665. When plague threatened the city in 1638, another Londoner remembered the epidemic of 1625 and how he had heard 'bells tolling and ringing out continually'.

In all these cases, with the notable exception of the Cheshire village, it is evident that some form of support for the sick and dying was attempted. Despite the flight of many members of the governing elite, civil and religious institutions were sufficiently resilient to keep some record of what was happening, and attempt to deal with the consequences. According to Boccaccio, people in Florence paid others to look after the sick and bury the dead, when they could afford it, and there emerged 'a kind of grave-digging fraternity, newly come into being and drawn from the lower orders of society'. Later on, these officers were financed by local rates, precarious though their income was when tax-payers disappeared. Among them were the women who acted as 'searchers' of the dead, distinguishing cases of plague from others as best they could, and 'bearers' or 'buriers', employed to carry the sick to plague hospitals or isolate them in their houses, and finally to carry them to their graves.

Often accused of making critical circumstances worse, these officers had a thankless task. Two of the bearers of the dead in

Florence in 1630 were accused of stealing a shirt off a corpse; they claimed it was a gift from the widow and that they had used it to cover another body. In the small English city of Salisbury in 1627, some of the bearers of the dead had to break into a house where everyone had died of plague: 'the smell of the house, with the heat of the infection, was so grievous they were not able to endure it'. Another bearer, a woman, had even been accused of burying people alive. A little girl had seen her coming with a winding sheet, and been heard to shout out, 'You shall not put me in a bag as you did my sister'. That may well have been malicious gossip, but plague necessarily had a brutalizing effect on all the parties involved. Those Salisbury bearers of the dead were found by the mayor of the city one night in the churchyard, 'dancing among the graves' and 'singing "Hey for more shoulder-work" in a fearful manner'.

That piece of drunken graveyard humour, almost a 'dance of death' in reality, was not unique. During epidemics in Avignon, there were dances among the graves in 1394, and searchers of the dead played leapfrog over corpses there in 1720. For those who had to do the dirty work, an intelligible response to the tensions imposed by death and sickness was to make mockery of them, just as it was for a man in York in 1632 'dancing and fiddling' among infected houses, or another who told an inquiring constable that all in his house 'were in health but his cat was sick'. These were some of the voices which take us beyond mere numbers and towards those 'sufferings of individuals' which Thucydides thought scarcely endurable.

Voices and victims

The sources from which the course and impact of epidemics can be reconstructed increased in variety over the period of the second pandemic. From the later 16th century, there were new genres of publication about plague, written by a wide spectrum of authors, from cardinals to cobblers, in vernacular languages more often than in Latin, and in verse as well as prose. They seem to have flourished first in Italy, during a series of epidemics between 1575 and 1578, and were then copied elsewhere. Some of them were accounts of the progress and outcomes of epidemics, which combined some of the qualities of the chronicles and plague tractates of the 14th and 15th centuries and added careful accounts of the origin and course of a particular epidemic. They were supplemented by shorter descriptions, by journals and occasionally diaries, by special forms of prayer against plague and thanksgivings for its departure, by semi-fictional stories, and by personal expressions of grief in verse, successors to the Welsh poems of the 14th century. A whole medley of different kinds of plague writing, varying in literary quality and purpose, and including some famous classics like Defoe's *Journal of the Plague Year*, originated in the later 16th century and in Italy.

Much of this literature was stimulated by policies for the control of plague which had also begun in Italy. They brought new players into the plague arena, in the shape of literate officials responsible for managing epidemics, who reported on their experiences and sometimes described them at length to inform their successors. One of the longest and most influential of the plague treatises of the 1570s was written by the chief medical officer of the kingdom of Sicily, appointed to take charge of public health there during the epidemic. Although a physician trained in the great medical school of Padua, he said little about cures for individual patients, but tracked the course of the disease and concentrated on the strategies of local magistrates, including quarantine measures, the separation of the sick from the healthy, and improvements to public hygiene, which might limit its spread.

None of this could be accomplished anywhere without opposition. Physicians in Padua itself argued that some of the epidemics of the 1570s were not 'true plague'; their findings had to be qualified or contradicted. Some public health measures interfered with the ceremonies of the Church by imposing limits on the numbers at funerals or in public processions in order to reduce the risk of infection; but in practice, Church authorities cooperated. The heroic exploits of Archbishop Carlo Borromeo among the infected of Milan in 1576–7 won him a reputation as lasting as that of Gregory the Great in Rome a thousand years earlier, but they included compromises about processions and public prayers: he encouraged people in quarantine to come to their windows to sing the Litany and hear Mass. During the same epidemic, a merchant from Alessandria trapped by plague in Milan wrote two plague tracts: the first attacking the 'great cruelty, avarice, iniquity, tyranny, vengeance, derision and theft' inflicted by local officers in the name of public health; the second—at the end of the epidemic—'congratulating' all the citizens on their endurance and even praising the servants of the health board appointed to visit houses and guard the gates 'who never became arrogant but diligently performed their duties'.

There were always two stories to tell about plague, one about heroes undeterred by contagion, the other about victims of harsh officialdom and of quarantine measures which might increase their exposure to infection by preventing any escape. The fullest accounts tried to combine the two and show men and women, physicians, churchmen, magistrates, and citizens trying to cooperate in impossible circumstances. In them, we begin to hear personal testimonies dominated not by unthinking panic or reckless bravado, but by courage in the face of overwhelming affliction. Most poignant of all are expressions of the pain and loss created by one of plague's cruellest features: the heavy mortality it inflicted on individual families and households, as relatives and servants died one after the other.

Some of them come to us at second hand, through court records and occasionally reported speech. There are many references to people left alone in infected houses when their relatives had perished, and forced when sickness overtook them to make their wills orally through windows to neighbours standing outside.

They were as strong-minded as the woman shut up in an infected hovel in Salisbury who told the mayor that 'my husband and two of my children cannot speak to me' and that she hoped for better days. In London in 1665, a schoolmaster found 'a poor woman who had buried some children of the plague' lying in a tiny room next to the open coffin of her husband; and another observer saw from his window 'a woman coming alone, and weeping by the door where I lived ... with a little coffin under her arm', on her way to the churchyard.

The sufferings of the illiterate majority can only be glimpsed indirectly, but those who were literate found ways of expressing their feelings, particularly about the death of children. An early example comes from a letter to Datini, the merchant of Prato, from a friend who had lost his wife and two children in an epidemic in Florence in 1400. 'Imagine how my heart broke', he writes, 'as I heard the little one weeping, and their mother not strong, and I heard the words of the eldest' child, who said 'he was called to judgement, and was ready to obey'. Three centuries later, similar statements survive in much greater number. During a plague in Barcelona in 1651, a tanner, Miquel Parets, recorded in his journal that he lost his wife, his two older sons, and a little daughter: 'she was like an angel, with a doll's face, comely, cheerful, pacific and quiet'. In a similar journal from Bologna in 1630, a glassmaker described how two of his daughters died, the youngest, an 8-year-old, raising eyes to heaven 'so bright and beautiful that she appeared not sick but well'. When his wife also died he stopped writing: 'May God rest her soul. I can write no more.' He died himself five days later.

Such accounts of grief are painful to read, but their circumstances testify to 'the travails and misfortunes and privations that are suffered wherever the plague is found, which are more than any person can stand', as Parets puts it. He tells us that his wife's two sisters refused to visit her in her sickness, 'as everyone fled from the plague'. Yet he thought it 'quite right to flee in order not to suffer from this disease'. He tells us about the lack of nurses for the sick, about their houses being nailed up, and about how some of them were carted off to pesthouses, but also about 'the good order and care of the district officials' and of the clergy who worked there. He tried to give a full account of this 'most cruel' disease, but found his pen inadequate to the task. 'I witnessed the many travails of many persons…so many that it would take a long time to tell it, but you should be able to imagine it thanks to what little I have…written.'

Hard choices

The fuller the sources become over time, the easier it is to test the accuracy of those sweeping statements of chroniclers about the havoc created by plague, and to see that the reality for everyone involved in an epidemic was personal stress. They had to weigh concern about their own safety and that of their families against the pull of other obligations and loyalties, inculcated by Christian morality or the everyday ties of friendship, business, and neighbourhood (see Figure 13). They faced hard choices. Datini of Prato was one of those perplexed by the issue of flight. His doctor, wife, and friends urged him to escape at the first sign of infection in Tuscany, but business affairs and scruples about deserting his employees held him back. In the end, in 1400, he fled from plague in Florence, and salved his conscience by signing a will on the day he left, giving most of his fortune to charitable purposes, 'for the love of God'.

Samuel Pepys, a man less susceptible to qualms of conscience than Datini, also found that making his will brought a 'much better state' to his soul in 1665, and faced similar practical problems. Detained in London by government business, he consulted the bills of mortality to judge the danger of infection in particular localities, noted its concentration in the poorest parishes, and kept away from infected houses and corpses in the street until he could no longer avoid them and 'came almost to think nothing' of such

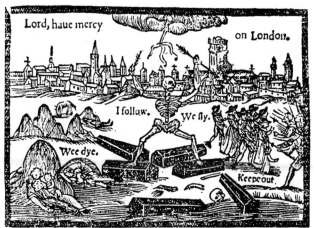

Lord, haue mercy   on London.

I follow.   We fly.

Wee dye.   Keepe out.

Printed at London for *Iohn Trundle*, and are to be sold at his Shop in Smithfield. 1625.

13. Death and flight outside the walls of London in 1625.

things, 'this disease making us more cruel to one another than dogs'. He moved his wife out of town to Woolwich early in July as soon as plague reached his own neighbourhood, and when his doctor died from it in late August and the quarantine of sick households seemed to have wholly broken down, he quickly joined her, going into London only when urgent business dictated.

Members of city councils and magistrates had greater local obligations, and were conscious of them. During a plague in Hull in 1637, an alderman sent his family out of town and would have joined them, he said, had he not been dissuaded by his concern for the citizens 'so sore visited' and by pressure from colleagues and local clergy. Many of his equivalents across Europe acted differently. From Seville to Florence and Milan to Moscow, large numbers of city councillors fled during epidemics, leaving behind a rump of dedicated men to impose what order they could. When the mayor of Exeter fled in 1625, one of his predecessors, Ignatius Jordan, filled the gap, appointing watchmen and distributing alms to the infected himself. He was careful not to 'causelessly expose himself to danger; yet being in the discharge of his duty he feared not the plague'. Jordan was a famous local Puritan, driven to action by religious convictions as fervent as those of Borromeo, the Catholic Cardinal of Counter-Reformation Milan.

Other clergy and members of religious orders were also subject to calls of duty which conflicted with obvious self-interest, and duty sometimes took second place. The Jesuits were famous for their dedication, visiting the sick, hearing their confessions, and organizing meals for them, street by street, in Rome in 1566. On occasion, they had to break down doors to get into houses, and found 'husband, wife, and children, more dead than alive, naked on the ground since they had not bed nor even a mat on which to lie'. When similar action in other cities led to their own colleges being quarantined, however, they became more cautious, even refusing a request from Borromeo in 1576 for volunteers to help him in the plague hospital of Milan. 'Although everyone must be ready to risk their lives to help the souls of others', one statement of Jesuit policy declared, each college must calculate the risk of exposing their members needlessly to infection, 'because sometimes you lose more than you gain in divine service'.

Survival for ordinary citizens marooned in a plague-stricken city similarly depended on cold calculation. They were daily faced with conflicting obligations to families, friends, and neighbours and, when it came to the point, not all ties of duty and charity were alike. As one 16th-century theologian explained, in an epidemic 'that which is not so near must give place to the nearer'. The servants of a household usually suffered most. A widow employed as a nurse in Essex in 1665 caught plague herself, and was left lying dead 'at least three days in the yard, at the mercy of hogs and dogs, most shamefully and unchristianly as the like never was heard'. As the language suggests, that was an exceptional case, but many sick servants were simply thrown out by their masters.

However, parents rarely treated their children, or children their parents, in the same way.

Other relatives were a different matter. Boccaccio's description of brothers abandoning brothers, 'uncles their nephews, sisters their brothers' in Florence in 1348 can be supported by cases in later outbreaks of plague, like the sisters who refused to visit Parets's wife in Barcelona. But such choices can rarely have been automatic, especially when close relatives lived under the same roof. In Salisbury in 1627, one householder turned his sister out of his house when she had plague, 'by which means, thanks be to God, I saved…the rest of my family': the decision, and others like it, left him 'overwhelmed with grief and perplexed on every side'.

Wherever they were enforced, quarantine regulations imposed exactly this kind of segregation and isolation on small families, but it is easy to forget that they were as often supported by people who wished to protect themselves and their children as they were opposed by those who found themselves shut up. When the inhabitants of some infected houses in York broke out of them in 1604, they were driven back by people in the next street, which was still free from plague. In 1603, a famous London astrologer, Simon Forman, packed a sick servant off to her family in Lambeth in order to prevent his house being shut up. Lambeth men sent her back again, saying it was better that Forman's household should 'starve and die, than any of them should be put in danger.'

The suffering of those subjected to strict quarantine, deprived of all freedom of movement, threatened by disease themselves, can readily be imagined, and can be documented at length from 17th-century court records and narratives by eye-witnesses. A printer in Malaga in 1649, for example, set out to describe 'a few of the endless number of pitiable cases in the city'. In one house, five children and two servants had died at home, and the father in the plague hospital 'where his mother (more than 60 years old) had come to take care of him'. In another, the mistress had died while nursing her baby and one of her elder daughters soon after, while she was feeding it; two other children died in the arms of African slaves employed to carry them to the pesthouse. The infant had been taken away to be looked after by 'a charitable woman'.

Nevertheless, people somehow learned to live and die with such privations, and even to accept the inevitable and put a brave face on it. A carpenter joining one of the processions organized by Borromeo in Milan in 1576 was told that officers of the city's board of health had shut up his house and shop. He replied calmly that he must first finish his prayers and would then 'shut myself up in my house in order to undergo quarantine'. Those employed to look after the sick in plague hospitals showed similar fortitude and resilience. The surgeon at the Saragossa pesthouse in 1653 had watched his wife and four servants die, and fell ill himself, but continued at his post 'working...without ceasing...taking care of the sick there', and survived. Another survivor was a surgeon in Augsburg who had lived and worked through several epidemics and never caught plague himself, and who deduced that medical practitioners and ministers of religion were 'protected above all others by Almighty God'. For people like him, faith in an ultimately beneficent providence promoted a selfless dedication to civic as well as religious duty.

Perhaps the most remarkable case in England comes from the small village of Eyam in Derbyshire in 1666, where the activism of the local parson, William Mompesson, became as renowned in later centuries as that of Borromeo in Milan. Mompesson kept his parish wholly isolated from others round about, no one being allowed in or out, with the result that nearly half his parishioners perished. It is probable that he was constrained to do so by pressure from outside. Local magistrates would otherwise not have supplied food and cash to the village. But he brought his own energy and confidence to the effort. When his wife died of plague he wrote to his patron 'the saddest letter that ever my pen did write, the destroying angel having taken up his quarters without my habitation'. Nonetheless, he had found 'God more good than ever I thought or imagined'. As with Borromeo and Jordan in Milan and Exeter, Mompesson's conviction that God's destroying angel had some purpose in a sinful world was a call to action, to purge whole communities of corruption, physical as well as moral, by means which included public health precautions as well as prayers.

In the course of the second pandemic, Europeans came to accept policies and practices for the control of plague which managed to reconcile secular prudence with religious piety. In many respects, that combination was peculiar to Christian Europe. Other religions and cultures had their own defences against the private horrors and public cruelties created by plague, including physicians, hospitals, and religious processions, and people faced similar hard choices, about flight for example. What they did not have—until Europeans came and imposed it on them—was the whole machinery of quarantine and forced isolation which had been developed in Europe between the 14th and 17th centuries. In order to understand that contrast and its implications, we need to look more closely at why plague policies were invented in the first place and what purposes they came to serve.

Chapter 5
Public health

The policies to control plague devised by Europeans had far-reaching historical consequences. Their novelty lay in the assumptions they carried with them about the responsibilities of governments. Public authorities must not only deal with the consequences of disease, relieve and support the sick, for example, and bury the dead, but attack its causes and means of transmission and so mitigate its impact; and the same principles could be applied to other diseases wherever and whenever they were identified. The obligation of governments to act to protect the public when epidemics threaten, even at the price of some limitations on private liberties, is something we now take for granted. But it was once a novelty as controversial as other extensions to the powers of governors have been. It had to be invented and accepted. Most of what we understand by public health, its basic rationale and ideology, was first formulated in the context of plague, and in the first decades of the second pandemic. If the history of plague has a wider significance, it lies in that achievement.

It was not achieved painlessly. Restraints on movement and public assemblies, and the isolation of individuals, households, and sometimes whole communities, involved financial costs as well as the human sufferings illustrated in Chapter 4; and the benefits they offered were always open to question. Nevertheless,

European governments invested in an armoury of weapons to combat plague, and they did so long before its causes were known with any certainty. They had few precedents to guide them, apart from traditional treatments of leprosy by means of isolation and ritual cleansing sanctioned in the Old Testament. They must have learned something also from empirical observation of the ways in which plague spread rapidly across space, from continent to continent, city to city, and house to house. Simple pragmatism probably explains the first known instance of something approaching plague control, in 640, during the first pandemic, when there were attempts to restrain the movement of merchants along roads leading out of plague-stricken Marseilles.

At the beginning of the second pandemic, however, basic defence mechanisms were elevated into a programme, a code of practice, with a bureaucracy to support it. During the Black Death in April 1348, and within a few days of one another, first Venice and then Florence set up special health commissions of leading citizens to deal with the crisis. Their main duty was the enforcement of existing sanitary laws, but the Florentine commissioners were to remove 'infected persons' from the streets along with 'all putrid matter' since they might cause 'a corruption or infection of the air'. Both cities tried to stop travellers coming from infected places and to isolate the goods they brought with them, and so did smaller towns in Tuscany, including Pistoia where there were also restrictions on the numbers attending funerals to try to prevent further infection.

Quarantine in the strict sense of the word came slightly later. It began in the former Venetian colony of Ragusa (now Dubrovnik) in 1377, when all travellers and their goods coming from outside were isolated for thirty days. The practice spread and began to be targeted at ships and travellers from ports known to be infected, and the period of isolation varied slightly from place to place. In 1383, Marseilles insisted upon the forty days which quarantine, referring originally to Lent, literally implied. Venice itself had a quarantine station on an island in the lagoon from 1423, called the 'old lazaretto' when a new one was added to supplement it in 1468. They were soon used to isolate victims of plague from within Venice, and became models for pesthouses and plague hospitals elsewhere which generally adopted a similar plan, with small cabins around a large open square, usually with their own church or chapel.

The Duchy of Milan, which had somehow escaped serious infection in 1348–9, more than caught up with its competitors in plague epidemics between 1374 and 1468, and became another model of best practice. Able to act more quickly and decisively than the councils of Tuscan and Venetian republics, the Visconti and Sforza dukes copied their health boards and gave them extra work to do. They ordered local hospitals to take in the infected, had temporary shacks and cabins thrown up for them outside the gates, and then had a special plague hospital built for them, the *Ospedale Maggiore*, in 1456. Milan was one of the first cities to try to identify the contacts of the sick, and have them segregated separately, shut up in their own homes. The dukes were also responsible for the first regular monitoring of public health, demanding notification of all illnesses and deaths in the city in 1399, and instituting the formal registration of deaths which became permanent practice in 1452.

Central to all this activity were systematic methods of surveillance and segregation. Actual and potential sources of infection must be identified and isolated to halt the progress of infection. The dukes of Milan took a personal interest in making sure that happened, even though physicians disagreed about whether the disease was contagious or not. Most of the members of the Milan College of Medicine believed that plague was caused primarily by a putrefaction of the humours of the individual patient and not by contact with another infected person. The ducal physicians disagreed, and some of them were authors of the earliest plague treatises to expound a theory of contagion. For them, as for their employers, there was no doubt that plague was spread by close contact with infected places, persons, and property. The contact might come via touch and breath or through the corrupted air, the miasma, which surrounded sites of infection, but in either case, action could be taken to prevent it.

By the end of the 15th century, therefore, both the mechanisms and the rationale of plague policies had been established. There were to be further disputes about whether plague was contagious, as in Padua in the 1570s. The details of policy also varied from situation to situation and from one epidemic to another. But the fundamentals of segregation and surveillance persisted until the end of plague in Europe. They were already familiar in Italy in 1486, when the first permanent health board, the *Sanità* of Venice, was established to implement them; and they were ready to be tried and tested further afield.

Trial and error

The diffusion of Italian practices occurred in piecemeal fashion over more than a century, and they were never adopted wholesale in a single package. The details have to be reconstructed from a succession of ordinances or regulations which refer to restrictions on movement from infected places or the isolation of the sick in hospitals or their own homes. There are early instances of more than one of these in ports, as in Barcelona in 1408 and 1451, Antwerp in 1450, and Rouen in 1512, for example, as one might expect given their exposure to infection, and to information about how it was controlled elsewhere. Autonomous or semi-autonomous cities, heavily dependent upon long-distance commerce over land, soon followed the example of their Italian peers. Augsburg had its first plague hospital in 1521, for example, and Lyons another by 1531.

Once the process had begun, the capital cities of larger states and their princes and parliaments quickly joined in. Plague ordinances were issued by the Duke of Burgundy in 1524, and by the *Parlement* of Paris in 1533. In the centralized monarchy of England, plague regulations began with a royal proclamation against 'contagious infections' in 1518, and led in 1578 to the first of a series of printed books of plague orders issued whenever the disease arrived. Deliberately aimed at copying the 'civility' of Italy, and influenced by advice from physicians trained in Padua, they were supported by punitive sanctions authorized by an Act of Parliament in 1604. It gave watchmen legal authority to use 'violence' to keep the infected shut up in their houses. Anyone with a plague sore found wandering in the company of others outside was guilty of felony and might be hanged. Anyone else going out could be whipped as a rogue. The statute's stated intent was 'the charitable relief and ordering of persons infected with the plague'.

By the early 17th century, when there were similar ordinances all over southern and western Europe, public order and public health were closely allied. A long report on plague, written in 1631 by the French physician of Charles I of England, opened with the resounding commonplace that 'order is the soul and life of all things' and described the practices essential for 'the public health of all'. It advocated multiple pesthouses, the strict segregation of the sick from their contacts, and boards of health with the 'absolute power' necessary to implement its recommendations. In France, there were similarly grandiose ambitions, advertised in a 'political and medical treatise' about plague published in 1647. As its title indicated, political considerations came first. Magistrates were now declared to be 'the true physicians of the people'; and when 'they were obliged to use draconian methods' to maintain public health, it had to be recognized that they did so 'for the preservation of the state' which must always 'prefer the general interest to the particular'.

Ordinances and exhortations were one thing, of course, their practical implementation quite another. Few cities and states had the resources to undertake every aspect of Italian best practice.

The segregation and support of the sick and their contacts in different places was rarely attempted outside Italy. Pesthouses were much more common but could never house all the infected in major epidemics, and even in Florence many of them had to be shut up at home. Household isolation itself could not be sustained for long during a major epidemic crisis and often had to be suspended in some of the worst-affected parishes of large cities. Yet compulsory isolation, that quintessentially draconian method of ensuring order in the name of public health, was fundamental to European policies everywhere.

It could not have been attempted at all in the face of popular hostility had it not had some public support, from people of property and influence anxious to protect themselves. From that point of view, one of the most important features of plague epidemics after the 14th century was their visible concentration among the poor. That created a social divide and, since plague sometimes leapt across it, a collective sense on one side of the threat to public health represented by the other. It is no accident that the introduction of plague policies in the 15th and 16th centuries went hand in hand with new laws and institutions designed to regulate the movement of beggars and paupers, and to isolate the most dangerous of them. Laws ostensibly promoting social welfare and public health were closely related. They were part of what was later called 'police', a term which embraced policy and regulation, and one which implied the imposition of order and control. Plague policies involved the exercise of power and advertised the extent of its ambition.

Plague policies also offered other kinds of reassurance to the literate and the better off. They gave them information which persuaded them that the disease might be understood and could be avoided even if not completely controlled. The registration of deaths begun in Milan in the 15th century had led in some cities to the compilation and publication of bills of mortality which showed people like Pepys which parishes of a town to avoid and when to leave. With the passage of time, they also allowed plague to be seen in its historical context. A printed broadsheet sold in London in 1665 displayed statistics about deaths in the seven 'modern' plagues in the city up to that time, so that their relative virulence could be compared (see Figure 14). Plague was ceasing to be a wholly unpredictable stroke of providence, and coming to be viewed objectively.

There were clear indications of that shift in some of the publications about plague which proliferated in Italy in the 1570s, and it had occurred in England by the 1670s. In 1662, John Graunt used the bills of mortality as material for the first statistical analysis of disease, and the first published exercise in historical demography. He pointed to the many regularities in the epidemiology of plague, including its rise and fall with the seasons of the year, and demonstrated that London's population had recovered within two years of even the greatest mortalities, thanks to migration from the countryside. A few years later, the political economist William Petty, Graunt's colleague in the Royal Society, calculated that the next epidemic would probably be less severe than that of 1665, especially if he was paid to introduce improved methods of quarantine, and he was ready to lay wagers to that effect. Fortunately for him, perhaps, the bet was never put to the test, but it shows a cool calculation about risks from plague which would have been inconceivable 300 years earlier, when the second pandemic began.

From the point of view of governors, information about the incidence of plague was essential if they were to know where quarantine and isolation should be applied, but unlikely to help very much once an epidemic had taken hold. Accurate information was equally vital to efforts to prevent plague arriving in the first place, however, and there draconian measures had a greater chance of success. The royal governor of Seville, the Count of Villar, was unable to control an epidemic in the city in 1581. Spurred on by missives from King Philip II, he took great care

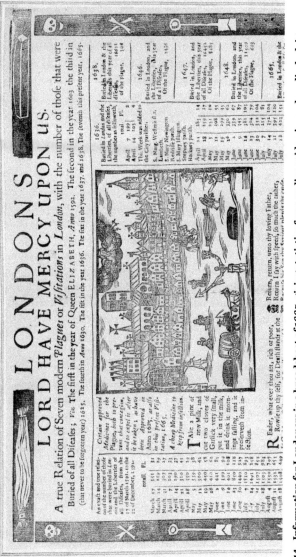

14. Information for Londoners in a broadsheet of 1665, giving statistics from earlier epidemics and medical advice alongside the illustration.

that it should not happen again, appointing commissioners to search for suspected cases in surrounding towns in 1582 and isolate them when they were identified. Thomas Wentworth, Charles I's president of the Council of the North in England, took similar action to protect York in 1631. What Wentworth called 'severe and strict courses' seem to have protected large cities on both occasions, though they might not have done. They failed when tried again outside Seville in 1599.

As suggested in Chapter 2 of this book, sanitary cordons on a much larger scale could be successful if the police action taken was strict and severe enough. The cordon which protected most of France from the plague in Marseilles in the 1720s involved one-quarter of the French standing army being stationed on the frontiers of Provence. As one historian remarks, it was 'one of the rather few occasions on which the absolutist state assumed powers that really were absolute'. The success of the long cordon between the Austro-Hungarian and Ottoman Empires in the 18th century similarly depended on military force. It was along a boundary policed initially for military defence, and the pay-off in terms of public health was secondary, but it was equally real.

The exposed ports along the sea coasts of the northern Mediterranean and western Europe had no such defences. Plague could only be kept at bay there by the successful quarantine of shipping from suspect harbours to the south and east, and that depended on more than local power and the insistence on bills of health from ports of origin. It required the exchange of accurate information on an international scale. Italian cities had again shown the way. In the 16th century, their boards of health had corresponded about the movement of infection, and in 1652 they tried to agree on a *concerto*, a convention for cooperation against plague.

That early gesture towards a World Health Organization failed. Systematic cooperation between states only began with the first

International Sanitary Conference in 1851, but long before then the great trading empires of Europe had their own information networks of agents and contacts which served a similar purpose. There were regular reports to London from the Baltic, when there was plague between 1708 and 1710, for example, and again from the Mediterranean in the early 1720s, when two suspect ships from Cyprus were quarantined and finally burned, parliament voting £24,000 as compensation to the owners. It was a price well worth paying for the kind of precautions which, when taken in scores of European ports, massively reduced the risk of plague returning.

It is therefore something of a paradox that at the very moment when plague was withdrawing from Europe, there should have been mounting scepticism about the efficacy of the plague precautions implemented once the disease arrived. It was during the last plague in England in 1665–6 that published criticism of household quarantine as wholly counterproductive was loudest, Graunt, among others, arguing that 'alterations in the air' were far more important causes of infection than 'contagion' between people. In 1708, a sanitary cordon around Königsberg erected by the Prussian government had to be removed in the face of local protests that it killed more people than the epidemic itself. The same point was made in Marseilles in the 1720s, when even one of the royal doctors asserted that he knew from experience that the disease was not contagious, and denounced the 'violence done to freedom' and the 'insults performed on people's rights' by the pretence that it was.

Scepticism about well-established policies was partly a result of the greater public knowledge and informed debate which came with the free flow of information. It was in tune also with the political and cultural climate of an Enlightenment Europe which was hostile to the exercise of absolute power, and confident about the benefits to be gained from local sanitary improvements which involved fewer threats to freedom of commerce and private liberties.

None of that undermined confidence in the need for public regulations of some kind for the protection of public health, however. The ambitions of 'medical police' were publicized at great length by J. P. Frank in the 1780s and continued to command assent. The defences of Europe against plague from outside also remained in place. If some commercial interests objected to their unnecessary rigour, others were increasingly aware of the dangers of plague coming in with imports of cotton. The quarantine of shipping was successful, and it was necessary because other parts of the world, closer to the sources of the disease, did not practise it.

Both points seemed obvious to some of the great figures of the Enlightenment. Looking back coolly over the centuries to the first pandemic, Edward Gibbon had no doubt about what was owed to 'those salutary precautions to which Europe is indebted for her safety'. Voltaire joined others in the general complaint about the 'Turkish fatalism' which supposedly inhibited Muslim countries from adopting quarantine, and thought it astonishing that people who were clever enough to have invented inoculation against smallpox should be so stupid that they ignored defences against plague which had proved their utility for so long. The plague policies of Europe were ripe for export to seemingly less enlightened continents.

Export

European conquerors and colonizers overseas took their version of public health with them, not as an incidental item in their baggage, but as an essential part of the civilizing mission which justified their imperialism. That was how it seemed to Spanish viceroys in the Americas like Villar, who went from Seville to Peru in 1585 and tried to attack smallpox and influenza epidemics as he had attacked plague back home. The outcome is not recorded, but control measures must have been met with the same hostility that his successors encountered from native populations which had no previous experience of European crowd diseases and little concept of contagion. The ground was better prepared for such innovation in the Muslim Mediterranean and the Persian Gulf, where plague and the quarantine precautions adopted by European powers were both well known, and where there were already pressures in the early 19th century for reforms along European lines.

The first signs of activism came in newly independent Greece and the more autonomous parts of the Balkans where there were at last *lazaretti* and quarantine stations, and in Egypt, thanks to the energy of Muhammad Ali, a modernizing pasha committed to what he called an 'ideology of order'. Having already set up a teaching hospital on the French model, in the 1830s he had sufferers from plague and their contacts isolated, and introduced sanitary cordons with battalions of troops ready to suppress all opposition. One of his French physicians, as critical of concepts of contagion as some of his contemporaries in Paris, was sceptical, and a British ambassador protested about the consequences for imperial commerce. The pasha was no more deterred than a 15th-century duke of Milan would have been in similar circumstances.

As this incident suggests, some European governments back home were losing confidence in draconian measures, which had proved unpopular and largely ineffectual when used against cholera. Even the quarantine laws which protected them against the import of plague were being modified, first in Britain in 1825 and then France in 1847, in order to allow local discretion in their implementation. In France, only Marseilles persisted with its previous severity— understandably, given the port's history. The British now considered sanitary cordons policed by troops characteristic only of 'rigorous military despotisms' like Russia, Prussia, and Austria, 'with their walled towns, and guards and gates'.

That left the British in something of a quandary, and open to the accusation of double standards, when their landed empire increased as fast as their overseas trade. They were opposed to the quarantine of shipping when it affected their own interests, and it needed international pressure in the 1860s to compel Britain to tighten up practices of quarantine in the ports of India so as to protect Europe from suspect goods shipped from there. When plague invaded their own dominions in the third pandemic, however, they were no less wedded to an ideology of local order than the pasha of Egypt. More than that, they made an imperial virtue of the fact. As an officer of the Indian Army Medical Service explained in 1898, 'plague operations ... properly undertaken' presented 'some of the best opportunities for riveting our rule in India' and 'also for showing the superiority of our western science and thoroughness'.

Thoroughness was the order of the day to begin with. It was first tested in Hong Kong in 1894 when plague arrived there from Canton, where local authorities provided doctors, hospitals, and medicines for the sick, but, as one European complained, 'no Sanitary Board, ... no sanitary or preventive measures, ... no isolation of cases'. All of these were introduced by the British government of Hong Kong, much to the dismay of the Chinese community. There were mass graves, streets walled up, and guards around them. When plague reached the crowded and more populous cities of India, there was panic on a scale unknown in outbreaks of cholera, though these had often been more lethal. All the private horrors of European plague were repeated across a whole subcontinent, and public policies imposed on thousands of victims by imperial power did little to mitigate them.

The government of India introduced a succession of regulations and new laws, including an Epidemic Diseases Act in 1897 which provided for plague committees in infected towns (see Figures 15 and 16). There were temporary plague hospitals and segregation camps, search parties tracked down plague cases, and infected houses were sometimes burned to the ground. In 1896, 100,000 Indians were reported to have fled from Bombay, 'precipitated by

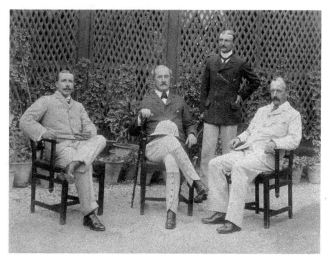

15. A committee charged with plague control in Karachi in 1897.

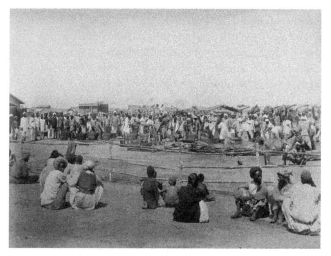

16. The Karachi segregation camp being disinfected (beyond the fence) in 1897.

compulsory hospitalization and the destruction of dwellings'. Eight out of ten of those taken to hospital died, and like Europeans centuries earlier, people preferred to be cared for by their relatives at home. Crowds attacked ambulances and stormed the plague hospital, and the local plague committee had to modify its policy. In Calcutta, compulsory segregation was abandoned in 1898 after similar riots and a mass exodus from the city. In smaller places, policy was sometimes more sensitive to Indian opinion, segregating victims by caste and religion, for example, but whole villages were nevertheless placed in quarantine, and there were still sanitary cordons and segregation camps years after they had been abandoned in Bombay.

In 1900, an Indian plague commission recommended an end to unduly repressive measures. It was one of a number of commissions trying to identify the causes and carriers of the disease, some of them sent out by European powers and including experts in epidemiology and bacteriology—Robert Koch among them. Several of their members came to think that plague was not communicable directly from person to person. Attention turned instead to rats, which were exterminated in their thousands despite opposition from Hindus, who believed all forms of animal life sacrosanct; and, when that proved ineffective, there were efforts to inoculate the contacts of plague victims, sometimes by force, which proved even more unpopular. In the absence of clear alternatives, the thorough segregation of plague victims remained the first British reaction to epidemics wherever they occurred. In Cape Town, South Africa, more than 6,000 Africans were moved out of town to shacks and barracks alongside a small plague hospital in 1900; and, in Sydney, Australia, a little later, 2,000 people were forced into a quarantine station and the many Chinese among them compulsorily vaccinated.

Racial prejudices were clearly involved in many of these colonial confrontations between policy and popular opinion, and the discriminatory incidence of plague certainly exacerbated them.

The social tension between those who were observed to be a source of infection and those who were threatened by it was the same as it had been in Europe, and so was the conclusion of governors that, in the words of a director-general of the Indian Medical Department, bubonic plague was 'a disease of filth, a disease of dirt, and a disease of poverty'. Just as in Europe, moreover, familiarity with the disease and its incidence in the end led Europeans themselves to question the necessity for draconian precautions and to relax their vigilance. By 1902, one of the British in India could say that Europeans were now 'indifferent' to plague, since 'the statistics show that fewer Europeans have died from plague than die each year from cholera, so we can chance plague as we chance cholera'.

Longer experience of the disease also changed opinion among educated non-Europeans, persuading many of them that there was much to be said in favour of state regulation of public health for reasons familiar from the European experience. Egypt had been an early example, as we have already seen, and when plague came to Alexandria again in 1899, a British government less securely established than it was in India received welcome support for plague controls from leaders of the Muslim community. 'Science and modernity were compatible with Islam', one of them roundly declared.

They were discovered to be compatible with imperial rule in China much more quickly. The late Qing regime could not ignore pressure from local reformers, European and Chinese, who were experimenting with quarantine. Neither could it ignore modernizing developments in Meiji Japan, which had adopted German concepts of state medicine and public health. When pneumonic plague hit Manchuria in 1910–11, it was prepared to react more aggressively than it had against bubonic plague in Canton in 1894. It set up a Plague Prevention Bureau in Shenyang, with a 'sanitary police' to control movement, examine houses for plague cases, and see them carried to isolation stations.

It singled out the poor for special attention, isolating them in wooden barracks and railway cars, since 'the cases of plague were largely restricted to the coolie class and the lowest orders'. The Russian administrators in Harbin and Fujidian, where nearly 10,000 people died, imposed similar controls, including mass cremations and forced quarantine.

They had some scientific justification for acting as they did. The foreign plague experts who descended on Manchuria as they had earlier flocked to India quickly established that they were dealing with a different and far more lethal form of the disease than the bubonic variety, and one which without any doubt passed directly from person to person. That scarcely justified the savagery with which they acted. In Manchuria, Qing and Romanov governors competed with one another to see which could most enthusiastically display what one historian accurately terms an 'imported modernity'.

Plague controls were imports, all the more alien to their victims because they were imposed lock, stock, and barrel in sudden bursts of sometimes brutal activity. They had been devised in Europe, not without difficulty, but over centuries. Before we conclude this chapter, we must ask why that should have been so.

Why Europe?

The question of why Europe was first with plague precautions is one part of the much larger issue of why Europe was first in a host of practices and institutions which contributed to 'modernity'. One approach to the question might be through the vast literature which has now accumulated on 'the rise of the West' and the 'great divergence' between West and East over the last few centuries. To pursue that avenue, however, would require a much larger book than this one and take us into complex and contested areas of scholarship, including disputes about relative standards of living across the globe and over time. It pays better dividends, and may make a modest contribution to that larger debate, if we stick close to plague and the policies adopted against it and look for particular reasons which account for one particular kind of divergence in the West. Even then, we are confronted with some large areas of uncertainty which have still to be properly investigated.

It is helpful first to emphasize precisely what it was that seemed both novel and wholly objectionable to the people and peoples who encountered plague regulations for the first time, whether in Europe or elsewhere. It was not the application of medical or quasi-medical theories to the treatment of disease. Throughout the Middle East, and in India and China, just as in Europe, people combined a belief in the supernatural origins of an epidemic disease, as the work of God or the gods, or of demons and spirits, with some secular interpretation of its natural aetiology, usually in terms of an imbalance in the constitution of those infected or some deficiency in the environment in which they lived. All of them had means of responding, which included prayers, processions and ceremonies, philanthropic support of those who were sick by communities or authorities, and treatment by learned physicians. Some of them used hospitals to house victims of infectious diseases, and, since they were familiar with leprosy as well as plague, had a rudimentary idea of contagion (unlike some native Americans). What they found offensive in the case of plague, however, were those practices of close surveillance and compulsory segregation that shattered community cohesion and violated the moral norms which sustained it.

That was not very different from the objections raised against plague policies by many Europeans who regarded plague as a threat to the whole community against which communal and not divisive defences should be employed. It was a matter of preserving the Christian values of charity and neighbourliness. European observers of epidemics in the Levant could not ignore the fact that Islamic societies were able to avoid some of the private horrors of plague common in Christian countries. According to a British surgeon in Aleppo in the 1790s, plagues were 'less terrible' in Turkish than in European cities because the markets were supplied throughout an epidemic, the sick were less likely to be wholly deserted, and the dead were decently buried, so that 'the dread of contagion' was 'much less prevalent' than in the West. When the government in Istanbul began to introduce sanitary precautions against plague in the 1830s, it opposed coercive forms of intervention like quarantines and confinement partly because in Islam plague was not a punishment but a reward for the faithful. It has been argued with respect to China similarly that powerful traditions of family, some of them rooted in the teaching of Confucius, militated against the ready acceptance of compulsory isolation there.

What is notable in Europe, however, is the way in which Christian ideals of charity proved less robust than equivalent value systems elsewhere. In Europe, religious leaders as different as Borromeo and Mompesson deferred to the secular power, or adopted its habits themselves, as they did in Rome. Christianity came to terms with secular interpretations of plague much more quickly than Islam or the various religions of China because of the pressure exercised on it by strong governments and magistrates. It would appear that it was not the content of particular moral or religious traditions which made the difference, but the relative power of religious and secular authorities in each context.

The reason why Europe was first in developing a particularly draconian code of public health seems likely to lie, therefore, in the realm of politics, and in some of the features which made western Europe different in its political make-up from the rest of the world, especially during the first two centuries of the second pandemic. In late medieval Europe, there were self-consciously competitive and ambitious cities and small states, not large amorphous empires. Some of them self-governing commercial entities and often ports, they observed plague being transported over sea and land, and had to respond. It was in the collective interest of Venice, Florence, Genoa, and Milan to take similar precautions, often in the face of medical opinion which denied that plague was contagious; and they had the will and resources to do so, by imposing wholesale quarantine and isolation.

The particular character of plague epidemics undoubtedly made its own contribution to the ways in which it was combated. It evidently came from outside, and its chief victims were the poor and disadvantaged, people with little political influence who seemed in need of control for other reasons. Surveillance and segregation followed naturally from that. Once begun, however, they appealed wherever rulers and regimes wanted to exercise greater control over their subjects, to develop and flex their bureaucratic muscles, and to ensure 'the preservation of the state', whether they were the would-be absolute monarchs of early modern Europe or the later governors of Egypt, China, and Japan who welcomed modernity. Plague policies and the notions of public health which they embodied were at root political constructs.

Chapter 6
Enduring images

The images that have been attached to plague are very diverse. They include graphic metaphors like the arrows of Apollo and the swords of biblical angels, which symbolize its causes; and literary conventions such as those of Thucydides and Boccaccio about the disruption of families and societies, which summarize its consequences. Over time, new icons have been added to them, such as plague-saints and plague-doctors; and metaphors were borrowed from other contexts and commonly applied to plague, like the Dance of Death and visions of the Apocalypse. Taken together, they determined how plague was imagined in the past and how it has been described in histories and fictions down to the present. Like the public health policies of Chapter 5, images of plague have a continuous history, invented and then elaborated over the centuries.

Invention and purpose

The earliest such images and the most long-lasting tell us about interpretations of plague quite distinct from the notions of contagion and local pollution which shaped the policies of governments. They referred to the supernatural causes of great epidemics, which, when properly understood and manipulated, similarly offered ways of driving the disease away. Many civilizations and religions have attributed disease, and epidemic disease in particular, to angry gods or spirits who must somehow be appeased, like the 'jinn' who wielded 'the sword of plague' in popular tradition in the Muslim world from the Middle Ages down to the 19th century. But no other religion has been as creative as Christianity in devising means of propitiating the gods through the use of intermediaries, notably saints specially identified for the purpose.

St Sebastian, martyred in the 3rd century, was the first of them. His association with plague began in 680 when his relics were brought from Rome to Parma and were said to have ended an outbreak of plague there. By the 16th century, there were pictures of him, his body shot through with arrows, in churches all over Catholic Europe. St Roch (or Rock or Rocco), pointing to a bubo on his thigh and sometimes shown with his dog, was often painted alongside him (see Figure 11). Roch was supposed to have been born in 1327, to have cured plague victims, and to have been fed by his dog in the woods after he caught the disease himself and was expelled from Piacenza. The date and the stories come only from sources in the early 15th century, however, when his cult originated and took off.

Other figures from the past were similarly resurrected and reinvented, their reputations usually beginning with the identification of some particular place to which they were attached and then spreading beyond it. Naples had the relics of St Gennaro (Januarius), a 4th-century martyr, including his miraculously liquefying blood which was carefully watched for omens of plague from 1527 onwards. Plague ended in Palermo in 1625 when the relics of St Rosalie, a 12th-century hermit, were carried in procession; and St Thecla, a 1st-century virgin, was supposed to have saved Este from plague in 1630. The Virgin Mary herself, the most universally popular of all intermediaries, was adopted by particular cities as their special protector, from Paris in the late 6th century to Venice and Lyons in the 17th. Often depicted in paintings and on processional banners shielding the citizens under her capacious mantle, she sometimes had Roch and Sebastian on either side of her.

Many of these images were *ex-voto* offerings, intended and believed to have instrumental effect. In the folk culture of pre-Reformation and Catholic Europe, the relationship between saints and those they specially defended was like that between patron and client or a feudal lord and his retainers. Popes like Urban VIII, who gave official approval to the cults of Rosalie and Roch in 1629, might not have put it so crudely, but it implied reciprocal duties and obligations almost of a contractual kind. Prayers and gifts to the saints certainly offered as much solace and hope of relief as the medicines bought from physicians or apothecaries, perhaps more. These were not passive responses to epidemics but a form of direct action, designed to gain some control by negotiation with the powers that sent them.

It followed from the reciprocity of the relationship that thanks must be given for mercies received, and the success of supernatural intervention commemorated, preferably in concrete or ritual form. Rome still has the statue of St Michael the Archangel sheathing his sword on Castel Sant'Angelo; Vienna, its plague monument on the Graben finished in 1693; and Budapest, a column in Buda and a chapel dedicated to St Roch in Pest commemorating epidemics between 1690 and 1711. In Venice, the churches of the Redentore and Santa Maria della Salute were built in thanksgiving for the departure of plague in 1576 and 1630 (see Figure 17), and there were votive processions to them, as well as to the Scuola of S. Rocco, in the regular ritual calendar of the doge and citizens. They are all reminders of the tenacious hold of religious perceptions of plague far into the 18th century—in Catholic Europe at least.

Graphic representations of plague, whether on monuments or canvas, often referred to more than its supernatural origin, however; and sometimes their only purpose can have been to

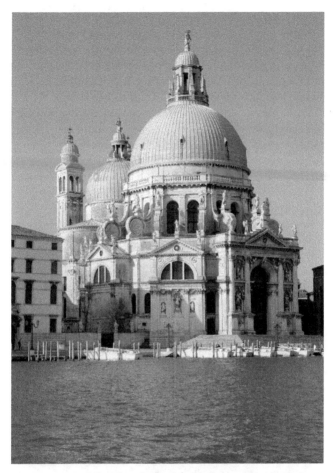

17. Santa Maria della Salute, built after the plague of 1630 in Venice.

show something of plague's reality. Several of the pictures of Carlo
Borromeo, which proliferated in oils, frescos, and engravings after
his canonization in 1610, show him ministering the sacraments to
the infected inside and outside the plague hospital of Milan in
1575–6, with images of the sick and dying all around him. There

are at least three contemporary paintings of the plague of 1656 in Naples, all of them focusing on the heaped-up bodies of the infected. They made as little reference to supernatural agencies as the early manuscript illumination showing coffins being hurriedly assembled which comes from Tournai during the Black Death (see Figures 5 and 7). Poussin's depiction of *The Plague of Ashdod* of 1630–1, which influenced many later artists (see Figure 18), refers back to the biblical plague of the Philistines and to their god, Dagon, who conspicuously failed them, but it seems chiefly designed to illustrate contemporary horrors wherever plague occurred. Prominent in the foreground is a representation of a dead or dying mother with a suckling infant, a motif whose origin lies in Raphael's drawing of *Il Morbetto*, itself much copied thanks to printed engravings derived from it.

By the 17th century, print was giving many kinds of images of plague a wide audience. Some of them were commissioned by

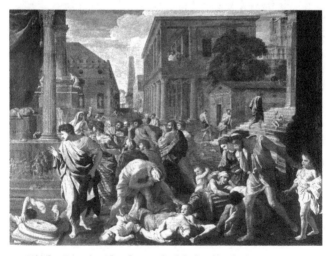

18. Nicolas Poussin, *The Plague of Ashdod*, painted 1630–1.

local authorities to present the official view of epidemics, and advertise the splendid modern precautions they adopted against them. There were engravings of new plague hospitals, but also of guarded gates and gallows for offenders against quarantine regulations, as in Rome during the plague of 1656–7. In the 1720s, the city of Marseilles commissioned prints which show a fine town hall and avenue leading to the pesthouse, but also bodies piled up on carts in front of them. Some of the earliest representations of plague-doctors, dressed head to foot in protective clothing and wearing masks with beaks containing aromatic substances, similarly, date from the plagues of the 1650s and 1720s, and can scarcely have been any more reassuring (see Figure 19).

Much cruder than any of these, and appealing to a more popular audience, were the woodcut illustrations of plague on cheap printed broadsides, which seem to have been particularly common in 17th-century London. One broadside shows several scenes in succession, as in a strip cartoon: a sick room with a searcher of the dead ready to examine the patient; streets with searchers, coffins, and funeral processions; the walls of the city, with corpses being buried outside them; and people in flight confronted by armed guards in the countryside. The intended effect was one of order being imposed amidst disorder, but it offered little hope of escape, only the necessity for resignation and endurance. Some of London's bills of mortality contained similar illustrations of the city, with a destroying angel or a triumphant skeleton like that in a dance of death alongside their statistics (see Figure 14). Other broadsheets recommended prayers as well as medicines to remind people of God's judgements, but in Protestant England, there could be no recourse to intermediaries and intercessors like the saints who might ensure some miraculous deliverance.

In London, as in some other cities, Catholic as well as Protestant, popular printed literature also offered ways of imagining plague in prose and verse as enduring as those on woodcuts and engravings. The plague pamphlets of Thomas Dekker published in England

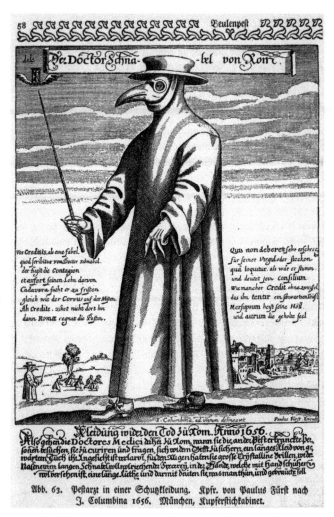

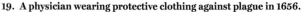

19. A physician wearing protective clothing against plague in 1656.

between 1603 and 1630 incorporated several of them. One had a title-page showing a plague-stricken London with an infant and dead mother in the foreground (see Figure 13) and its contents refer to Apollo and God's arrows striking the city's 'sinfully polluted suburbs'. Others called Londoners to repentance and condemned the way countrymen treated those who fled. But they also contained stories designed to amuse as well as to edify, like one about a drunkard waking up in a plague pit and finding himself surrounded by corpses. Dekker said he intended to evoke 'a happy laugh' in his readers because, as physicians had explained, 'mirth is both physical and wholesome against the plague'.

Satire, making fun of plague, was one way of fighting it, making it familiar, perhaps cutting it down to size. It had been used in the past, by a Florentine poet in 1532, for example, and was often to be used again, even by authors personally affected by the disease. Dekker's contemporary, Ben Jonson, depicted plague in what might seem to us wholly contradictory ways. In his plays, there are comical figures who bring plague in from London's suburbs, and a great projector, Sir Politic Would-Be, who hopes to make a fortune from his invention of special bellows to blow the smell of onions over ships in quarantine. Yet Jonson was also the author of a lament on the loss of his son, 'his best piece of poetry', who had died in the London plague of 1603. Jonson himself was safe in the country, where he had a vision of the boy with 'the mark of a bloody cross on his forehead', like the crosses on infected houses, and he blamed himself for this judgement of providence because he had loved his son too much.

When plague withdrew from Europe in the 18th century, it left behind multiple ways of representing it. Many of them were represented in the literature published in the 1720s and 1730s, in the wake of what turned out to be the last epidemic in France. There were narratives and medical tracts, odes and epistles, about the plague of Marseilles, including Jean-Baptiste Bertrand's *Relation historique*, written in 1721 while disease still raged there.

Along with drawings and engravings, they made the city itself an icon of plague for centuries after. Their equivalent in England was a single work, with a lasting influence all its own, Daniel Defoe's *Journal of the Plague Year*, published in 1722.

Defoe had reported on events in Marseilles in his newspapers, and he set out to reconstruct the London epidemic of 1665, with all its events 'public as well as private', in order to show what might happen again if the disease reached England from Provence. He drew upon publications from 1665 and had his narrator, 'H.F.', reflect on topics which were commonplace in earlier plague literature: the question of whether keeping plague secret in order to avoid panic was better than public knowledge of an outbreak; the vexed problem of flight; and the difference between proper religious piety in the face of infection and passive 'Turkish fatalism'. He reported stories which might easily have come from Dekker's pen or from accounts of earlier epidemics, about bearers of the dead suspected of stealing sheets off the backs of the corpses they buried, and about drunkards in alehouses mocking devout mourners outside and 'laughing at the word judgement'. But Defoe was particularly intrigued by the question of how far the interests of public safety should be allowed to override those of private individuals.

He had no doubt that plague was contagious, though others denied it. One of his newspaper reports shows that he had no time for the merchants who opposed quarantine restrictions on commerce, and in doing so ventured 'the welfare of the whole kingdom ... for the wretched gain of a private man'. In the *Journal*, he similarly defended household quarantine in London: 'It was a public good that justified the private mischief.' Equally, however, 'the severity of those confinements' made people desperate and disorderly. Defoe tried to understand both sides and not to condemn either of them. The actions of parish officers were sometimes 'cruel and rigorous', but they 'did their duties in general with as much courage as any, and perhaps with more', since they worked 'among the poor who were more subject to be infected and in the most pitiful plight'. All of them were victims of circumstance. 'There was no remedy: self preservation obliged the people to those severities which they would not otherwise have been concerned in.'

The comprehensive scope and balanced judgements of Defoe's *Journal* did as much as the quantity of publications about Marseilles to ensure that literary depictions of plague survived along with other images of what it had once meant. Like the Athens of Thucydides and Boccaccio's Florence in previous centuries, London in 1665 and Marseilles in 1720 became obvious points of reference when plague stimulated the imaginations of European authors again and old images were revisited after 1800.

Survival and revival

Memories of plague survived its disappearance from Europe in a variety of forms. Some of them were simply anachronisms, like the painting which Napoleon commissioned of his visit to the plague sick in a hospital in Jaffa in 1799, showing him in the role of another Borromeo. British cartoonists mocked his presumption. The need for intercessors and intermediaries was disappearing. But other images of plague were given a fresh vitality, the more distant they became from everyday experience. That was partly prompted by the perennial fascination of something wholly 'other', but interest in past plagues also gained a new relevance when cholera in the 19th century and HIV/AIDS and new virus infections in the 20th threatened to recreate similar epidemic disasters. Images and stories of plague in various literary genres acquired a life of their own.

The first indication of new life came just before or soon after Napoleon had himself painted as Borromeo, in the period between the 1790s and the 1830s. Before then, some images of plague, including metaphors of pollution and references to punishing deities, had been applied to smallpox, but that disease was more easily visualized as an individual affliction than as a sudden universal calamity. It encouraged a fascination with personal pain and the grief of the bereaved better suited to 18th-century sensibilities than recollection of collective horrors. Scares about 'pestilential fevers' spreading from the poor to the rich were sometimes revived by gaol fever, typhus, but cases were localized and irregular. Much closer to the real thing were outbreaks of yellow fever in North America in the 1790s and cholera in Europe in the early 1830s, which were as corrosive of some of the optimistic assumptions of the Enlightenment as the political disturbances and revolutions with which they coincided.

Cholera in particular evoked memories of plague. Histories of past epidemics had been published in New England in the 1790s, prompted by yellow fever. Cholera produced more, some of them popular, some of them founded on serious scholarship. Defoe's *Journal* was reprinted in full in 1835, for the first time since 1755, and with a modernized text. Hecker's seminal history of the Black Death appeared in 1832, and inaugurated a series of depictions of 14th-century epidemics, with their flagellants, dancing manias, and persecutions of the Jews, all of them examples of extremes of human behaviour scarcely acknowledged by the civilized sensibilities of the Enlightenment. Plague became a topic for 'Gothic' recreations of more barbarous ages, of disastrous events supposedly reshaping the whole course of history.

Changes in literary culture associated with Romanticism belong to the same period and also had their effect. It can be seen in the evolution of an image often associated earlier with plague and collective horror, the *danse macabre* (see Figure 8). It had been a part of folk culture since the 15th century, and given wide circulation by prints copying Holbein's famous drawings of 1538. In 1813, Goethe's poem *Der Totentanz* elevated the Dance of Death to literary prominence. His dancers, 'so poor and so young, so old and so rich', retained much of the social symbolism they had in the past, but the motif was soon put to new uses. It was employed by critics of the bourgeoisie and absolute government in 1848, and scenes of dances and balls allowed writers from Flaubert to Strindberg to explore more profound and intimate relationships between the living and the dead. The dance inspired musicians too, from Liszt or perhaps Schubert (in 'Death and the Maiden') onwards, and it acquired its own scholarly literature, beginning as early as 1826.

With or without a dance, plague itself became a popular topic for literary fiction in the early 19th century. The fashion began with a verse drama, John Wilson's *The City of the Plague*, published in 1816. Its dying heroine, from 'among the hills of Westmorland' and set against a contrasting background of plague-infected London, owes a good deal to the early Romantic poets, whom Wilson knew, but some of his scenes look back to much earlier literature. There is a satirical street party, for example, when the Master of the Revels, having lost his wife and mother in the epidemic, sings a 'Song on the Plague' in praise of 'the Pest'. Of little literary merit in itself, Wilson's macabre melodrama would have been wholly forgotten had its theme not appealed to others. It was read by Pushkin in 1830, when cholera raged throughout Russia, and was the basis for his short tragedy *The Feast in the Time of Plague*, published in 1832, which had many imitators. Feasts and revels became common settings for fictions about disease and mortality, including some deliberate horror stories like Edgar Allan Poe's *Masque of the Red Death* (1842) in which pestilence was material for nightmare rather than romance or social commentary.

Wilson's *City* also caught the interest of writers less distinguished than Pushkin in England. It prompted John Holland in 1821 to produce his own epic poem about the Derbyshire village of Eyam, which the local rector, William Mompesson, had isolated during the plague of 1666 (see Chapter 4). The poem had notes quoting Mompesson's letters, and inspired other publications which gave the village its reputation as a site of historic and heroic deeds and romance. After the bicentenary of the epidemic in 1866, Eyam became something of a tourist trap, complete with its own invented traditions, and in its small way a local version of Marseilles. Marseilles scarcely needed invented traditions when it commemorated the centenary of its own plague in the 1820s. The publications of the 1720s were reread, and historical records edited and published. They were nonetheless material for fiction, beginning in 1828 with Gilbert de Pixérécourt's 'historical melodrama' in three acts, *La Peste de Marseilles*, which has heroic young doctors, evil body-snatchers, and a pair of lovers at risk in a quarantined city.

The first modern novel about plague, and the first Italian novel of all, had been published in the previous year, 1827. Alessandro Manzoni's *The Betrothed* was a melodrama on a similar romantic theme, but it also had an extraordinarily accurate historical background, in this case the plague of Milan in 1629–30, whose detailed depiction takes up a large part of the book. Like the plays of Wilson and Pixérécourt, it owes something to Defoe, and contains vignettes not far removed from the historical record, including some bearers and buriers of the dead singing 'Long live the plague, and death to the rabble', just like the real bearers of the dead in Salisbury back in 1627. Other historical novels of a similar kind soon followed. One of the most popular, Harrison Ainsworth's *Old St Paul's* (1841), about the plague and fire of London, has a coffin-maker singing a 'song of the plague' with a toast for his customers: 'Drink the Plague! Drink the Plague!'

Despite their historical references and the research that lay behind them, Ainsworth's novel and some of its successors were very far from being accurate representations of plague in the 17th or earlier centuries. They reflected impressions of epidemics, whether Gothic or romantic, melodramatic or macabre, manufactured in the 19th century by the literary tastes and for the literate audience of the time. They were images as far removed from the reality as the disease was from European experience. In the 20th century, the distance grew even wider as literary fashions changed and educated readers responded to different, perhaps more demanding, kinds of fiction. Many novels about plagues and pestilences displayed little interest in history, sometimes dispensing with it altogether, and concentrated more self-consciously on what epidemics had to say about current anxieties and the human condition at the time.

The change of emphasis can be illustrated by a film, a fiction which exploited graphic as well as narrative images in a famous evocation of the Black Death, Ingmar Bergman's *The Seventh Seal* made in 1957. With its game of chess between Death and the Knight dominating the plot, and a final iconic dance of death driving home its message, the film might be regarded as the supreme embodiment of a Gothic view of the Middle Ages, when crusaders and peasants fought in vain against pestilence in a harsh and cruel environment. Its historical chronology is certainly confused, and its image of some ill-defined medieval century one of unrelieved and unrealistic gloom. Yet Bergman set out to create a parable not a chronicle. His title refers to the seventh seal in the Book of Revelation whose breaking is followed by a 'silence in heaven', by the Last Judgement, and by the end of the world. Its story is a moral fable for a modern nuclear age about the impossibility of sustaining religious faith, perhaps any kind of faith, in the face of imminent disaster.

Some of the reasons for using plague in this allegorical way were explained in an essay on 'The Theatre and the Plague' written in 1934 by Antoine Artaud, inventor of the 'Theatre of Cruelty' and a native of Marseilles who knew its history. He visualized plagues and theatrical performances as occasions for the exhibition of extreme forms of expression and action, and the ventilation of normally 'dormant images' and 'latent disorder'. One can readily see the appeal of the extreme to some of the authors of fictions in the 19th century, and the exploration of those dormant images has been much more prominent in plague literature since then. The disease has become established as a frame through which to view things other than plague itself.

Fiction and representation

There is nothing very new about the use of plague as a backdrop, creating a suitably threatening atmosphere and adding tension to a tale in order to point a moral. The plague of Athens serves that function for Thucydides. Boccaccio's description of the Black Death at the beginning of the *Decameron* hangs over the fictions which follow as a reminder of mutability and mortality. Plague provides an appropriate setting for an old story about drunkards finding death as well as gold under a tree in Geoffrey Chaucer's 'Pardoner's Tale'; and for a parable about political power and social injustice in La Fontaine's 17th-century fable 'The Animals Sick of the Plague'. While plague stories continue to have allegorical uses and moral purposes, however, the invention of the novel as a vehicle for the exploration of individual motivation and social interaction gave them greater scope to probe the strengths and weaknesses of individuals and social institutions subjected to exceptional stress.

In the past century, there has been a host of novels, and films based on novels, about epidemics—past, present, and future—all of them experimenting with stereotypical images and incidents familiar from earlier representations. One or two have become acknowledged classics of their kind, like Thomas Mann's *Death in Venice* (1912), Sinclair Lewis's *Martin Arrowsmith* (1925), and Katherine Anne Porter's *Pale Horse, Pale Rider* (1939). Each of them centres on the self-perception of an individual in a personal tragedy created by an epidemic, and all three present images of whole societies on the verge of dissolution. Philip Roth's *Nemesis* (2010) similarly deals with the personal crises of its central figure, a playground supervisor trying to do his duty to the children in his charge during a polio outbreak in 1944, and when he finally leaves, taking the 'arrow' of the disease with him and thereby 'scapegoating himself'. It is a narrative about his feelings of failure and eventually despair in a world abandoned by God, and also an allegory of the Holocaust, since many of the polio victims are Jews.

The list could easily be extended, and might embrace a great diversity of fictions. Sometimes titles refer directly to plague, as with Jim Crace's novel *The Pesthouse* (2007), about efforts to escape pestilence and famine in a future dystopian USA; or the horror film *Quarantine* (2008), describing the impact of a newly discovered or manufactured virus in a single apartment block. Jean Giono's *The Horseman on the Roof* (1951) uses some of the Marseilles literature in its story about cholera in Provence in 1832, and its title, like those of Bergman and Porter, is another deliberate reference to the apocalyptic prophecies in the Book of Revelation about the end of the world. A recent novel in Chinese, *Snow Raven* (2008) by Chi Zijian, seems to be unique in taking for its historical setting an epidemic of pneumonic plague, in Harbin in 1910–11, and has a range of characters reminiscent of some older European tales of plague and some modern stories about that and other kinds of disaster: a profiteering Japanese businessman, a Russian diva, a righteous local gentleman, and a Chinese doctor sent to 'save' the city.

Stories of this kind have multiple functions whose exploration would take us far away from plague, and so do images of the disease which flourish in other recent genres of popular culture, from zombie fictions to video games. All of them no doubt have a cathartic effect, raising emotional temperatures and tension, and relieving them in a process as therapeutic as Dekker hoped a reading of his plague pamphlets would be. They may evoke terror or excitement, and have something to say about ourselves, our personal and collective anxieties. If they repay the attention of students of plague, however, it is because they convey as vividly as Defoe's *Journal* how people were compelled to behave when plague was a real and not merely an imagined phenomenon. Images of plague can be manipulated in a variety of ways, but the best plague fictions have successfully evoked the historical character of epidemic situations.

From that point of view, Albert Camus's *The Plague* (1947) still stands as the pre-eminent example of the genre. Set during an imagined plague epidemic in the port of Oran in North Africa in the 1940s, it can be read as an allegory, about French resistance to Nazi oppression, or about inescapable and arbitrary evil in a world as meaningless as Bergman's. It owes much to Defoe and the published accounts of plague in Marseilles; and it explores personal dilemmas as moving as those depicted by Roth and a range of actors as various as those of Chi Zijian. Like many of its successors, it also recreates the personal and collective dilemmas which plague posed in the past and which were illustrated in Chapters 4 and 5 of this book: the hard choices which had to be faced in impossible circumstances and the ways in which the actions of authority aggravated them, not needlessly but necessarily.

Camus's narrator, Dr Rieux, finds himself a 'prisoner of the plague' along with everyone else when Oran is placed under quarantine and no one allowed to leave. Conventional religion begins to lose its hold, superstitions and rumours abound, and there is 'much heavy drinking'. Long-established communal ties are shattered, and men and women compelled 'to live, as individuals, in relative solitude'. 'None could count on any help from his neighbour; each had to bear the load of his troubles alone.' Rieux has his own problems. As a doctor 'watching men dying who were meant to live', his task was 'no longer to cure, but to diagnose. To detect, to see, to register and then condemn.' In his narrative, however, he seeks to take 'the victims' side' and share with them 'the only certitudes they had in common—love, exile and suffering'. 'There was no predicament of theirs that was not his.'

The predicaments are those inevitable in plague-time and illustrated through his friends. Among them are Paneloux, a Catholic priest, energetically doing his religious duty, exposing himself to infection in hospitals and outside, until in the end even he has religious doubts about a beneficent divinity; and Cottard, a criminal obsessed with trying to escape but 'the living image of content' for a time, as he profits from plague by selling drink and tobacco at inflated prices. There is Richard, another physician, denying that plague is plague at the beginning of the epidemic; and Rambert, a journalist, wanting to escape to rejoin his lover in Paris, but finally understanding that everyone is engaged in a common struggle and he must stay to retain his self-respect. Closest to a hero perhaps is Grand, the municipal clerk, organizing the work of sanitary teams disinfecting houses, keeping registers of deaths and sickness, and trying and failing to get beyond the first sentence of a fiction he is composing, about a woman on a pale horse (an apocalyptic image again). For Grand, unlike some of the others, there is no point in trying to comprehend plague or find any meaning in it. It is enough to know that 'plague is here and we've got to make a stand; that's obvious'.

In the end, Rieux takes a similar standpoint. He has no doubt that restrictions on movement are essential in the interest of public health: the question is not whether the measures taken are too 'rigorous, but whether they are needful to prevent the death of half the population. All the rest is administrative action.' At the same time, however, he intends his chronicle to 'bear witness in favour of those plague-stricken people; so that some memorial of the injustice and outrage done them might endure; and to state quite simply what we learn in a time of pestilence: that there are more things to admire in men than to despise'. Defoe's narrator might have said much the same thing. Central to Camus's novel as to all histories and stories about plague is that persistent tension between the individual and the community, between private and public interests, which is created by epidemic disease itself and by the precautions that have to be taken against it.

There is also another theme common to accounts of plague, past as well as present. Many of them refer to the difficulty of creating any literary representation of plague which encompasses every aspect of it and allows the reader to comprehend the whole. Rieux confesses that he is no more successful at that than his friends who keep their own records. Parets, the Barcelona tanner recording the plague of 1651 in Barcelona, knew that there was much more to be said than his simple prose could express; and Mompesson's letters from Eyam acknowledge that he is describing something that exceeds 'all history and example'.

A combination of history and fiction might be thought most likely to succeed, and it has been attempted. Manzoni, the pioneering Italian novelist, undertook historical research for the purpose in 1827; and John Hatcher, an eminent medieval historian, uses 'creative reconstructions' of character and dialogue 'far closer to docudrama than conventional history' in *The Black Death: An Intimate History* (2008). Yet the mass of historical detail sometimes overwhelms much of the plot of the first; and the comparative success of the second is achieved only by avoiding plot and presenting 'a sequence of set pieces' which illuminate much of what the Black Death meant at the time but not, of course, the whole.

Narratives about plague can no more provide a complete image of their subject than pictures of saints or engravings of infected cities. They will always be inadequate. But we must try to draw other lessons from histories of plague before we can conclude this very short and inadequate introduction.

Chapter 7
The lessons of histories

Different kinds of histories of plague, in different genres, have been introduced in this book. Some have been serious works of medical science or historical scholarship, others narratives by contemporaries who experienced the disease at first hand, or fictions drawing to a greater or lesser degree on earlier testimonies. All have had their own voices and their own ways of framing a complex reality. Mine has been a historian's view of them, designed to show how they were all shaped by the circumstances in which they were created and the audiences they addressed, and all, in consequence, in one way or another incomplete. I have tried to show also how much they had in common in the topics and themes they dealt with, and the questions they raised. Despite their diversity of voice and approach, they were talking about the same thing.

It is striking how narratives about plague, whether histories or novels, contemporary chronicles or reports to governments and their agents, have all focused on the same issues: on the dilemmas faced by individuals trapped by infection; on attempts at control which attacked contagion between places and the pollution of particular local environments almost in the same breath; and on ways of imagining plagues which offered or denied the prospect of salvation from them. Even the very different medical and historical debates about the aetiology and epidemiology of plague have engaged two sides with much in common. There is no dispute about the fact that plague appeared in different forms in different centuries; that the pathogen responsible evolved and continues to evolve over time, albeit very slowly; and that more than one species of rodent and flea has had a role in its transmission. Those modern historians who have argued that *Yersinia pestis* cannot have been responsible for the Black Death, and those who think the great weight of the evidence, especially the evidence of ancient DNA, points the other way, have both been looking at the same phenomenon and disputing only one element in it. There has been considerable continuity over the centuries in the ways in which plague epidemics have been experienced, combated, described, and argued about.

Treating plague as a single topic can also be justified because it set a pattern, a template, for the ways in which other epidemic diseases were represented and treated when they first appeared. In the 14th century, when it was aggravated by other environmental shocks, plague itself had seemed to be a wholly exogenous phenomenon, an autonomous agent shaping its own history in ways people were powerless to influence. After that, however, the incidence and extent of plague mortality on any particular occasion were determined, and seen to be determined, by the context in which they occurred, by local conditions which dictated how quickly the disease moved and where it took root. Its character was influenced also by how people responded, sometimes more or less instinctively, by flight, for example, sometimes more deliberately by trying in one way or another to control it. Whether they were effective or not (and I have suggested earlier that they sometimes were effective), the quarantine policies invented and developed in early modern Europe demonstrated the role played by political cultures and political institutions in shaping reactions to plague.

It is scarcely surprising that other epidemic diseases were treated, at least initially, in the same way. The same tools were quickly used against cholera in Europe in the 19th century; and on a global scale against influenza in the great pandemic of 1918–20, when there were quarantine orders of every kind across the world, from Canada to Australia. In parts of the USA there was 'a thicket of ordinances' regulating behaviour and imposing social distancing in order to combat the disease. After 1920 it was the experience of the great flu as well as the history of plague that shaped responses to new or 're-emerging' diseases which seemed to threaten fresh pandemic disasters. HIV/AIDS is a famous example, provoking alarm about a new plague when first identified in California in 1981, and still a serious cause of morbidity and mortality in areas of the world where it is endemic. Other virus infections, like Marburg and Lassa fever, were identified as potential threats to the developed world at much the same time; and since the 1990s there have been further 'new' diseases causing similar anxieties, like SARS (severe acute respiratory syndrome), which appeared to be a new disease when it hit Toronto in 2003, and was subsequently discovered to have come from south China via Hong Kong. Before the arrival of COVID-19 there had been new strains of influenza occasioning similar scares, like 'H5N1', identified first in Hong Kong in 1997, and perhaps coming again from south China; and 'H1N1', identified in 2009 in Mexico. Both thought to be related to 'bird flu' or 'swine flu', they prompted the slaughter of poultry in suspected foci of infection, like the slaughter of rats during plagues in India a century earlier.

On their first appearance, each of these has been greeted in the press as a 'coming plague', and thought likely, given the speed of modern transport and the rapid mutation of viruses, to cause pandemics on a global scale. In 2019, Corona-virus proved to be exactly that. It spread across the world in a few months; and the speed of modern communications also meant the rapid adoption of common weapons aimed at controlling it. They included all the tools first invented and developed for control of plague and then used again in 1918–20, notably quarantine and the isolation of victims and their contacts, and restrictions on travel across borders; and as with plague precautions in 17th-century Italy, they were copied from one country to another in a competitive process as one state tried to prove itself more effective, more in command of events, than the rest.

Just as in the 17th century too, governments and their advisers have tried to measure their success or failure over time. Mathematical techniques have been employed as means of surveillance and monitoring far more sophisticated than the registration of plague deaths in bills of mortality in the seventeenth and eighteenth centuries, but with the same purpose—to bring the authority and order of numbers to superficially random events. In the 1660s John Graunt was the first to see the potential for detailed analysis of plague presented by the London bills. He searched for equivalent data from cities elsewhere so that he could analyse when and where plague mortalities were greatest, and he was able, with the limited evidence at his disposal, to suggest that epidemics were commonly more severe—but of shorter duration—in southern than northern Europe. His modern successors are the mathematical modellers who have calculated recent rates of infection in outbreaks of influenza, compared equivalent data over time, and produced projections of what might happen in future outbreaks if they are not halted when first identified.

Models have also been used to measure the likely efficacy of various forms of intervention should some future virus emerge and generate an epidemic explosion. The most important lesson to be drawn from them is one which would have been wholly familiar to people fighting plague in the past: that it is essential, wherever possible, to catch the first cases, and to isolate them before any epidemic occurs. In the case of a fast moving, highly infectious viral disease, that is much easier said than done, of course. But if it fails, nothing is certain.

In 2006, a group from Imperial College (later involved in advising the UK government on COVID-19) published a paper in *Nature* on 'Strategies for Mitigating an Influenza Pandemic'. It estimated the potential success of different policies and provided an accurate forecast of what was to come:

> We find that border restrictions and/or internal travel restrictions are unlikely to delay spread by more than 2–3 weeks unless more than 99% effective. School closure during the peak of a pandemic can reduce peak attack rates by up to 40%, but has little impact on overall attack rates, whereas case isolation or household quarantine could have a significant impact, if feasible.

The paper contained another reflection which throws light on past as well as present experience. It acknowledged that its model took no account of the behavioural changes which would occur once an epidemic had begun, and reduce rates of infection by increasing the social distance between clinical cases, members of the same household, and people outside it. There are certainly many examples of people in the past who distanced themselves in one way or another from plague, like the Londoners in 1625 who had been advised to keep at least two yards away from people they met in the street. But there are just as many instances of people deliberately ignoring rules restricting numbers at funerals in plague-time (no more than six in London in 1603), or going to the alehouse instead. Models may be useful guides for modern policy-makers, but their projections are not infallible predictions, and their authors know that they are scarcely more likely to get future outcomes right than the rulers of Milan, Venice, and Florence who first fought plague with new tools 500 years ago.

Fortunately COVID-19 has not proved to be as serious in terms of mortality as the influenza epidemic of 1918–20 which killed an estimated fifty million people across the globe; or the plagues of the 14th century which between them cut the population of Europe by at least a third. It is highly infectious but case-fatality rates have been very low. That is not, of course, to underrate the very much larger impact in the short and medium term of the costs of providing for a sudden reduction in economic activity and productivity. No one can tell whether the next new viral infection will be equally or far less benign. All that historians can say about future pandemics, if they are not snuffed out quickly by medical or political interventions, is that public and private responses to them will be necessary, diverse, and divisive, and no more certain to succeed than they were in the past.

As for the plague strategies adopted in previous centuries, it is impossible to pass any final judgement on the rights and wrongs of control policies which involved so many costs and such uncertain benefits. The historian can only echo what Camus makes his narrator, Dr Rieux, conclude in *The Plague*. Rieux knew that 'the plague bacillus never dies, or disappears for good' and that the 'tale he had to tell could not be one of a final victory. It could be only the record of what had had to be done, and what assuredly would have to be done again' by people who refuse 'to bow down to pestilences'.

Histories of plague have only modest lessons to offer. They tell us about the importance of cultures and institutions, contexts and agents, in creating epidemics and reactions to them. They show that the ways in which people think and live, the kinds of information available to them, and the kinds of behaviour they adopt—to flee, or to fight, or simply to be fatalistic—make a difference. But they hold out no prospect of painless victory once an epidemic has begun. We might give the last word to Daniel Defoe, reflecting on the personal afflictions and public terrors in a plague year: against them, he says, 'there was no remedy'.

References

References are given here for statements and quotations whose sources are not readily identifiable in the books in the Further Reading section.

Chapter 1: Plague: what's in a name?

Plague and biological terrorism: David T. Dennis, 'Plague as a Biological Weapon', in I. W. Fong and Kenneth Alibek (eds.), *Bioterrorism and Infectious Agents: A New Dilemma for the 21st Century* (New York: Springer, 2005), pp. 37–65.

Nutton on the biological agent of the Black Death: Vivian Nutton (ed.), *Pestilential Complexities: Understanding Medieval Plague* (London: Wellcome Trust, 2008), p. 16.

Papers of 2010 on microbiological and archaeological evidence: G. Morelli et al., '*Yersinia pestis* genome sequencing identifies patterns of global phylogenetic diversity', *Nature Genetics*, 42 (2010): 1140–3; S. Haensch et al., 'Distinct clones of *Yersinia pestis* caused the Black Death', *Public Library of Science, Pathogens*, 6 (2010): 10.

Rosenberg: Charles E. Rosenberg, *Explaining Epidemics and Other Studies in the History of Medicine* (Cambridge: Cambridge University Press, 1992), pp. 306–7.

Chapter 2: Pandemics and epidemics

Climatic shocks: Bruce M. S. Campbell, 'Nature as historical protagonist: environment and society in pre-industrial England', *Economic History Review*, 63 (2010): 281–314.

Kazakhstan: N. C. Stenseth et al., 'Plague: past, present and future', *Public Library of Science, Medicine*, 5 (2008): 1.

Boccaccio: Rosemary Horrox, *The Black Death* (Manchester: Manchester University Press, 1994), pp. 26–7.

Explanations for the disappearance of plague in the 18th century: A. B. Appleby, 'The disappearance of plague: a continuing puzzle'; Paul Slack, 'An alternative view', *Economic History Review*, 2nd series, 33 (1980): 161–73 and 34 (1981): 469–76; Edward A. Eckert, 'The retreat of plague from central Europe, 1640–1720: a geomedical approach', *Bulletin of the History of Medicine*, 74 (2000): 1–28.

Austrian sanitary cordon: Gunther E. Rothenburg, 'The Austrian sanitary cordon and the control of the bubonic plague, 1710–1871', *Journal of the History of Medicine*, 28 (1973): 15–23; Daniel Panzac, *Quarantaines et Lazarets. L'Europe et la peste d'Orient* (Aix-en-Provence: Édisud, 1986), pp. 79–102.

Gregory of Tours: Lester K. Little (ed.), *Plague and the End of Antiquity* (Cambridge: Cambridge University Press, 2007), p. 11.

Chapter 3: Big impacts: the Black Death

'Too much else going on': Peregrine Horden, 'Mediterranean plague in the Age of Justinian', in Michael Maas (ed.), *The Cambridge Companion to the Age of Justinian* (Cambridge: Cambridge University Press, 2005), p. 156.

Villani: David Herlihy, *The Black Death and the Transformation of the West* (Cambridge, MA: Harvard University Press, 1997), pp. 47–9.

Sicily and Tuscany: S. R. Epstein, 'Cities, regions and the late medieval crisis: Sicily and Tuscany compared', *Past and Present*, 130 (February 1991): 3–50.

Flanders and Holland: Bas van Bavel, *Manors and Markets: Economy and Society in the Low Countries 500–1600* (Oxford: Oxford University Press, 2010), p. 87.

England and France: Christopher Dyer, *An Age of Transition? Economy and Society in England in the Later Middle Ages* (Oxford: Oxford University Press, 2005), pp. 156–7, 235.

Hecker: J. F. C. Hecker, *The Epidemics of the Middle Ages* (London: Sydenham Society, 1844), p. 32.

Gasquet: Francis Aidan Gasquet, *The Great Pestilence* (London: Simpkin Marshall, 1893), p. xvi.

Meiss: Millard Meiss, *Painting in Florence and Siena after the Black Death* (Princeton, NJ: Princeton University Press, 1951), p. 61.

Pogroms: Samuel K. Cohn, Jr, 'The Black Death and the burning of Jews', *Past and Present*, 196 (August 2007): 3–36.

Marseilles: Daniel Lord Smail, 'Accommodating plague in medieval Marseilles', *Continuity and Change*, 11 (1996): 13.

Cohn: Samuel K. Cohn, Jr, *The Black Death Transformed* (London: Arnold, 2002), pp. 228–38, 244.

Chapter 4: Private horrors

Thucydides: Thucydides, *The Peloponnesian War*, tr. Rex Warner (Harmondsworth: Penguin Classics, 1954), pp. 123–9.

Boccaccio: Rosemary Horrox, *The Black Death* (Manchester: Manchester University Press, 1994), pp. 28–34.

Pepys: Robert Latham and William Matthews (eds.), *The Diary of Samuel Pepys*, 11 vols (London: G. Bell and Sons, 1970–83), vi, pp. 189, 201, 256.

Chapter 5: Public health

Milan: Ann G. Carmichael, 'Contagion theory and contagion practice in fifteenth-century Milan', *Renaissance Quarterly*, 44 (1991): 213–56.

Grandiose ambitions of French absolutism: Colin Jones, 'Plague and its metaphors in early modern France', *Representations*, 53 (1996): 97, 116, 118.

Graunt and Petty: John Graunt, *Natural and Political Observations... upon the Bills of Mortality* (London, 1662), pp. 36, 38, 41; Marquis of Lansdowne (ed.), *The Petty Papers*, 2 vols (London: Constable, 1927), i, p. 26.

Gibbon: Edward Gibbon, *The Decline and Fall of the Roman Empire*, Everyman edn. (London: J. M. Dent, 1910), pp. iv, 373.

Voltaire: Voltaire, *Oeuvres complètes*, ed. Louis Moland (Paris: Garnier, 1877–85), vol. xxix, p. 304.

Turkish fatalism: Nükhet Varlik, '"Oriental plague" or epidemiological orientalism', in Varlik, ed., *Plague and Contagion in the Islamic Mediterranean* (Newark: ARC Humanities Press, 2017), pp. 57–88.

'Indifference' to plague in India, 1902: Rajnarayan Chandavarkar, 'Plague panic and epidemic politics in India, 1896–1914', in

Terence Ranger and Paul Slack (eds.), *Epidemics and Ideas* (Cambridge: Cambridge University Press, 1992), p. 209.

'Science and modernity' in Egypt: William Beinart and Lotte Hughes (eds.), *Environment and Empire* (Oxford: Oxford University Press, 2007), p. 180.

'Imported modernity' in Manchuria: Mark Gamsa, 'The epidemic of pneumonic plague in Manchuria 1910–11', *Past and Present*, 190 (February 2006): 168.

Literature on the 'Rise of the West' includes: W. H. McNeill, *The Rise of the West* (Chicago: University of Chicago Press, 1963); Kenneth Pomeranz, *The Great Divergence* (Princeton: Princeton University Press, 2000).

Plague less terrible in Aleppo: Patrick Russell, *The Natural History of Aleppo* (London: G. G. and J. Robinson, 1794), vol. ii, pp. 338–9.

Religious or cultural differences: Carol Benedict, *Bubonic Plague in Nineteenth-Century China* (Stanford, CA: Stanford University Press, 1996), pp. 127–8; Michael W. Dols, *The Black Death in the Middle East* (Princeton: Princeton University Press, 1977), pp. 297–301; Nükhet Varlik, '"Oriental plague" or epidemiological orientalism', in Varlik, ed., *Plague and Contagion in the Islamic Mediterranean* (Newark: ARC Humanities Press, 2017), pp. 57–88.

Chapter 6: Enduring images

Plague saints: Gauvin Bailey et al., *Hope and Healing: Painting in Italy in a Time of Plague, 1550–1800* (Worcester, MA: Clark University, 2005), pp. 21, 32, 191, 201, 229; Louise Marshall, 'Manipulating the sacred: image and plague in Renaissance Italy', *Renaissance Quarterly*, 47 (1994): 488–9, 503.

Tournai illustration: Joseph Polzer, 'Aspects of fourteenth-century iconography of death and plague', in Daniel Williman (ed.), *The Black Death: The Impact of the Fourteenth-Century Plague* (Binghamton, NY: Centre for Medieval and Early Renaissance Studies, 1982), p. 111.

Poussin and Raphael: Gauvin Bailey et al., *Hope and Healing: Painting in Italy in a Time of Plague, 1550–1800* (Worcester, MA: Clark University, 2005), p. 227.

Dekker: F. P. Wilson (ed.), *The Plague Pamphlets of Thomas Dekker* (Oxford: Oxford University Press, 1925), pp. 31, 135.

Jonson: Ernest B. Gilman, *Plague Writing in Early Modern England* (Chicago: University of Chicago Press, 2009), pp. 131, 163, 172.

Bertrand: Daniel Gordon, 'The city and the plague in the Age of Enlightenment', in *Yale French Studies*, 92, *Exploring the Conversible World*, ed. Elena Russo (New Haven, CT: Yale University Press, 1997), pp. 77–81.

Defoe: quotations taken from Daniel Defoe, *A Journal of the Plague Year*, ed. Louis Landa (Oxford: Oxford University Press, 1969).

Dance of Death: Sarah Webster Goodwin, *Kitsch and Culture* (New York: Garland, 1988), pp. 3–4, 13, 18, 64; Rudolph Binion, *Past Impersonal: Group Process in Human History* (DeKalb, IL: Northern Illinois University Press, 2005), pp. 136–7.

Wilson: Daniel Gordon, 'The city and the plague in the Age of Enlightenment', in *Yale French Studies*, 92, *Exploring the Conversible World*, ed. Elena Russo (New Haven, CT: Yale University Press, 1997), pp. 94–6.

Eyam: Patrick Wallis, 'A dreadful heritage: interpreting epidemic disease at Eyam, 1666–2000', *History Workshop Journal*, 61 (Spring 2006): 40–50.

Marseilles centenary, Manzoni and Ainsworth: David Steel, 'Plague writing: from Boccaccio to Camus', *Journal of European Studies*, 11 (1981): 96–100.

Artaud: Daniel Gordon, 'The city and the plague in the Age of Enlightenment', in *Yale French Studies*, 92, *Exploring the Conversible World*, ed. Elena Russo (New Haven, CT: Yale University Press, 1997), pp. 77–8.

Camus: for quotations from *La Peste*, I have used the English translation, Albert Camus, *The Plague*, tr. Stuart Gilbert (Harmondsworth: Penguin, 1960).

Chapter 7: The lessons of histories

Pandemic of 1918–20: Samuel K. Cohn, *Epidemics* (Oxford: Oxford University Press, 2018), pp. 441–4.

New diseases since 1980: D. Ann Herring and Alan C. Swedlund (eds.), *Plagues and Epidemics* (Oxford: Berg, 2010), pp. 1–2, 29, 179.

Comparison with plague precautions in Italy: Guido Alfani and Tommy Murphy, 'Plague and lethal epidemics in the pre-industrial world', *Journal of Economic History*, 77 (2017), pp. 336–7.

Paper in *Nature* (2006): Neil M. Ferguson et al., 'Strategies for mitigating an influenza pandemic', *Nature*, 442 (27 July 2006): 448–52.

Camus and Defoe: Albert Camus, *The Plague*, tr. Stuart Gilbert (Harmondsworth: Penguin, 1960), pp. 251–2; Daniel Defoe, *A Journal of the Plague Year*, ed. Louis Landa (Oxford: Oxford University Press, 1969), p. 152.

Further reading

General works

There is no up-to-date overview of plague across the centuries, but
there are some stimulating surveys of disease and history more
generally, especially William H. McNeill, *Plagues and Peoples*
(Oxford: Blackwell, 1977), and for more recent periods, Sheldon
Watts, *Epidemics and History: Disease, Power and Imperialism*
(New Haven: Yale University Press, 1997); Peter Baldwin,
Contagion and the State in Europe, 1830–1930 (Cambridge:
Cambridge University Press, 1999); and Mark Harrison,
Contagion: How Commerce Has Spread Disease (New Haven: Yale
University Press, 2012). Christian W. McMillen's *Pandemics. A
Very Short Introduction* (Oxford: OUP, 2016) is an excellent
account of a large topic.

For an introduction to different approaches to epidemic disease in the
past, see Charles E. Rosenberg, *Explaining Epidemics and Other
Studies in the History of Medicine* (Cambridge: Cambridge
University Press, 1992); D. Ann Herring and Alan C. Swedlund
(eds.), *Plagues and Epidemics: Infected Spaces Past and Present*
(Oxford: Berg, 2010); and the essays in Terence Ranger and Paul
Slack (eds.), *Epidemics and Ideas: Essays on the Historical
Perception of Pestilence* (Cambridge: Cambridge University
Press, 1992).

On the history of plague itself, the best guides to controversial areas
are the essays in Vivian Nutton (ed.), *Pestilential Complexities:
Understanding Medieval Plague* (Medical History, Supplement
no. 27, London: Wellcome Trust, 2008). Some relevant articles and

papers will be found in the References section of this book. Two works in French are full of indispensable information: Jean-Nöel Biraben, *Les hommes et la peste en France et dans les pays européens et méditerranéens*, 2 vols (Paris: Mouton, 1975–6), and Daniel Panzac, *La Peste dans l'Empire Ottoman 1700–1850* (Louvain: Peeters, 1985).

The disease

General summaries can be found in G. C. Cook and Alimuddin I. Zumla (eds.), *Manson's Tropical Diseases*, 22nd edn. (Edinburgh: Saunders/Elsevier, 2009); and Kenneth F. Kiple (ed.), *The Cambridge World History of Human Disease* (Cambridge: Cambridge University Press, 1993). Thomas Butler, *Plague and Other Yersinia Infections* (New York: Plenum Medical, 1983) is a modern description; and L. Fabian Hirst, *The Conquest of Plague: A Study of the Evolution of Epidemiology* (Oxford: Oxford University Press, 1953), a classic, though now somewhat dated, account by another author who knew the disease at first hand. Books throwing doubt on the identity of plague in medieval and early modern Europe are: Graham Twigg, *The Black Death: A Biological Reappraisal* (London: Batsford, 1984); and Susan Scott and Christopher J. Duncan, *Biology of Plagues: Evidence from Historical Populations* (Cambridge: Cambridge University Press, 2001). Their scepticism is comprehensively challenged by Ole J. Benedictow, *What Disease Was Plague? On the Controversy over the Microbiological Identity of Plague Epidemics of the Past* (Leiden: Brill, 2010). For examples of important recent research on the ancient DNA of plague, see especially Monica H. Green, 'The Four Black Deaths', *American Historical Review*, 125 (2020): 1606–31; and also Maria A. Spyrou et al., 'A phylogeography of the second plague pandemic revealed through analysis of historical *Yersinia pestis* genomes', *Nature Communications*, 10/4470 (2019); and Barbara Bramanti et al., 'The third plague pandemic in Europe', *Proceedings of the Royal Society, B.*, 286: 20182429, 115/50 (17 April 2019): 11790–7.

The Plague of Justinian

Lester K. Little (ed.), *Plague and the End of Antiquity: The Pandemic of 541–750* (Cambridge: Cambridge University Press, 2007) is an indispensable collection. A more popular account is William Rosen, *Justinian's Flea: Plague, Empire and the Birth of Europe* (London: Pimlico, 2006).

The Black Death

There have been many books about the Black Death since J. F. C. Hecker's *The Epidemics of the Middle Ages*, tr. B. G. Babington (London: Sydenham Society, 1844). Philip Ziegler, *The Black Death* (London: Collins, 1969) remains useful as a general introduction. William Naphy and Andrew Spicer, *The Black Death and the History of Plagues* (Stroud: Tempus, 2000) is well illustrated and covers a longer period. Rosemary Horrox, *The Black Death* (Manchester: Manchester University Press, 1994) is a useful collection of source materials.

The best modern scholarly works are, for originality, Samuel K. Cohn, Jr, *The Black Death Transformed: Disease and Culture in Early Renaissance Europe* (London: Arnold, 2002); and for thoroughness of detail, Ole J. Benedictow, *The Black Death 1346–1353: The Complete History* (Woodbridge: Boydell, 2004).

There is important material on the Middle East in Michael W. Dols, *The Black Death in the Middle East* (Princeton: Princeton University Press, 1977); and Nükhet Varlik, *Plague and Empire in the Early Modern Mediterranean World: The Ottoman Experience, 1347–1600* (Cambridge: Cambridge University Press, 2015). There is much of general interest also in David Herlihy, *The Black Death and the Transformation of the West* (Cambridge, MA: Harvard University Press, 1997), which concentrates on Italian material.

Some of the most interesting recent work, particularly on the economic history of the period, concentrates on England. The essays in Mark Ormrod and Phillip Lindley (eds.), *The Black Death in England* (Stamford: Paul Watkins, 1996) cover a lot of ground comprehensively; and John Hatcher and Mark Bailey, *Modelling the Middle Ages: The History and Theory of England's Economic Development* (Oxford: Oxford University Press, 2001) is a splendidly sustained argument about the importance of plague. Hatcher has taken the theme forward into the 15th century, summarized in his *Plague, Population and the English Economy 1348–1530* (London: Macmillan, 1977), and given it imaginative as well as scholarly treatment in *The Black Death: An Intimate History* (London: Weidenfeld and Nicolson, 2008).

Plague in Europe, 1400–1800

Italian sources have provided material for some excellent books, especially Samuel K. Cohn, Jr, *Cultures of Plague: Medical Thinking at the End of the Renaissance* (Oxford: Oxford University Press, 2010); Ann G. Carmichael, *Plague and the Poor in Renaissance Florence* (Cambridge: Cambridge University Press, 1986); and Carlo M. Cipolla, *Public Health and the Medical Profession in the Renaissance* (Cambridge: Cambridge University Press, 1976). John Henderson's *Florence Under Siege: Surviving Plague in an Early Modern City* (New Haven: Yale University Press, 2019) is a thorough and rewarding account of a plague in 1630–3. On Venice, see Jane Stevens Crawshaw, *Plague Hospitals: Public Health for the City in Early Modern Venice* (London: Routledge, 2012).

Paul Slack, *The Impact of Plague in Tudor and Stuart England* (London: Routledge and Kegan Paul, 1985) covers similar ground for England; and J. F. D. Shrewsbury, *A History of Bubonic Plague in the British Isles* (Cambridge: Cambridge University Press, 1970) is strong on the chronology of epidemics, but less reliable in some of its conclusions. The best of several books on the 1665 epidemic in London is A. Lloyd Moote and Dorothy C. Moote, *The Great Plague: The Story of London's Most Deadly Year* (Baltimore: Johns Hopkins University Press, 2004); and there is an excellent account of an epidemic in Newcastle in Keith Wrightson, *Ralph Tailor's Summer: A Scrivener, His City and the Plague* (London: Yale University Press, 2011). Reactions to one Spanish plague are well described in Alexandra Parma Cook and Noble David Cook, *The Plague Files: Crisis Management in Sixteenth-Century Seville* (Baton Rouge: Louisiana State University Press, 2009); and to another in Ruth Mackay, *Life in a Time of Pestilence. The Great Castilian Plague of 1596–1601* (Cambridge: Cambridge University Press, 2019).

There is material on French reactions in Laurence Brockliss and Colin Jones, *The Medical World of Early Modern France* (Oxford: Oxford University Press, 1997); and on Russia in John T. Alexander, *Bubonic Plague in Early Modern Russia: Public Health and Urban Disaster* (Baltimore: Johns Hopkins University Press, 1980). Edward A. Eckert, *The Structure of Plagues and Pestilences in Early Modern Europe: Central Europe, 1560–1640* (Basel: Karger, 1996) and Lars Walløe, *Plague and Population: Norway 1350–1750*

(Oslo: Det Norske Videnskaps-Akademi, 1995) focus more heavily on epidemiology and demography. Karl-Erik Frandsen, *The Last Plague in the Baltic Region, 1709–13* (Copenhagen: Museum Tusculanum Press, 2010) is useful on epidemics in the North.

William G. Naphy, *Plagues, Poisons and Potions: Plague-Spreading Conspiracies in the Western Alps c. 1530–1640* (Manchester: Manchester University Press, 2002) is a detailed study of plague scares, a subject considered over a much wider canvas in Samuel K. Cohn, *Epidemics. Hate and Compassion from the Plague of Athens to AIDS* (Oxford: Oxford University Press, 2018). Important books on quarantine are Daniel Panzac, *Quarantaines et Lazarets. L'Europe et la peste d'Orient* (Aix-en-Provence: Édisud, 1986) and Alex Chase-Levenson, *The Yellow Flag: Quarantine and the British Mediterranean World* (Cambridge: Cambridge University Press, 2020), which can be supplemented by John Booker, *Maritime Quarantine: The British Experience, c. 1650–1900* (London: Ashgate, 2007). There are vivid first-hand accounts of plague in the letters of Francesco Datini, cited in Iris Origo, *The Merchant of Prato: Daily Life in a Medieval Italian City* (London: Penguin, 1963), and in the later sources used in Giulia Calvi, *Histories of a Plague Year: The Social and the Imaginary in Baroque Florence* (Berkeley, CA: University of California Press, 1989); James S. Amelang, *A Journal of the Plague Year: The Diary of the Barcelona Tanner Miquel Parets 1651* (New York: Oxford University Press, 1991); and A. Lynn Martin, *Plague? Jesuit Accounts of Epidemic Disease in the 16th Century* (Kirksville, MO: Sixteenth Century Journal, 1996).

Plague outside Europe

Plague in the Middle East has attracted some valuable scholarly work in recent years. In addition to the works of Dols and Panzac mentioned above, see Yaron Ayalon, *Natural Disasters in the Ottoman Empire: Plague, Famine, and other Misfortunes* (Cambridge: Cambridge University Press, 2015); and Nükhet Varlik, ed., *Plague and Contagion in the Islamic Mediterranean* (Newark, NJ: ARC Humanities Press, 2017).

The history of plague in China and India before 1800 remains to be written. Carol Benedict, *Bubonic Plague in Nineteenth-Century China* (Stanford, CA: Stanford University Press, 1996) is therefore a path-breaking book, and it can usefully be compared and contrasted with the account of plague-free Japan in Ann Bowman Jannetta's *Epidemics and Mortality in Early Modern Japan* (Princeton: Princeton University Press, 1987).

British India has understandably been better served, especially by Mark Harrison, *Public Health in British India: Preventive Medicine 1859–1914* (Cambridge: Cambridge University Press, 1994); and David Arnold, *Colonizing the Body: State Medicine and Epidemic Disease in Nineteenth-Century British India* (Berkeley, CA: University of California Press, 1993). The chapter on 'Plague and Urban Environments' in William Beinart and Lotte Hughes, *Environment and Empire* (Oxford: Oxford University Press, 2007) covers the whole of the British Empire in commendably succinct fashion.

Plague in art and literature

The Black Death has again stimulated a large amount of work on plague's cultural and artistic impact. Daniel Williman (ed.), *The Black Death: The Impact of the Fourteenth-Century Plague* (Binghamton, NY: Center for Medieval and Early Renaissance Studies, 1982) is a useful collection; and Samuel K. Cohn, Jr, analyses cultural reactions in *The Cult of Remembrance and the Black Death: Six Renaissance Cities in Central Italy* (Baltimore: Johns Hopkins University Press, 1992). Among many discussions of images of death and the macabre, Paul Binski, *Medieval Death: Ritual and Representation* (London: British Museum Press, 1996) is particularly perceptive and well illustrated. Christine M. Boeckl, *Images of Plague and Pestilence. Iconography and Iconology* (Kirksville, MO: Truman State University Press, 2000) takes the theme into the modern period.

Millard Meiss, *Painting in Florence and Siena after the Black Death* (Princeton: Princeton University Press, 1951) is a classic and now much criticized interpretation. Diana Norman, *Siena, Florence, and Padua: Art, Society and Religion 1280–1400* (New Haven: Yale University Press, 1995) is a useful corrective. Gauvin Bailey, Pamela Jones, Franco Mormando, and Thomas Worcester, *Hope and Healing: Painting in Italy in a Time of Plague, 1550–1800* (Worcester, MA: Clark University, 2005) is a well-illustrated catalogue with much of interest to say about the uses of artistic and architectural representations after 1500.

Plague

English literary responses to plague between 1500 and 1700 have been
material for several books, including Ernest B. Gilman, *Plague
Writing in Early Modern England* (Chicago: University of Chicago
Press, 2009). For European literature about plague after it
disappeared, two useful studies are Sarah Webster Goodwin,
*Kitsch and Culture: The Dance of Death in Nineteenth-Century
Literature and Graphic Arts* (New York: Garland, 1988); and
Barbara Fass Leavy, *To Blight with Plague: Studies in a Literary
Theme* (New York: New York University Press, 1992).

Daniel Defoe's *Journal of the Plague Year* and Albert Camus's *The
Plague* are, naturally, discussed in the books just cited, but anyone
interested in plague will want to read the works themselves.

Index

For the benefit of digital users, indexed terms that span two pages
(e.g., 52–53) may, on occasion, appear on only one of those pages.

Plague